DO NOT REMOVE
CARDS FROM POCKET

7/20/93

Combating Your Child's Cholesterol

A Pediatrician Shows You How

Combating Your Child's Cholesterol

A Pediatrician Shows You How

Reuben Reiman, M.D.
with
John Hanc

With a Foreword by
William P. Castelli, M.D.

Plenum Press • New York and London

Library of Congress Cataloging-in-Publication Data

Reiman, Reuben.
    Combating your child's cholesterol : a pediatrician shows you how
/ Reuben Reiman, with John Hanc.
        p.   cm.
    Includes bibliographical references and index.
    ISBN 0-306-44468-2
    1. Hypercholesteremia in children--Prevention. 2. Atherosclerosis
in children--Prevention. 3. Low cholesterol diet.   I. Hanc, John.
II. Title.
RJ399.H94R45   1993
618.92'3997--dc20   92-43287
                                                                          CIP

ISBN 0-306-44468-2

© 1993 Reuben Reiman and John Hanc
Plenum Press is a division of Plenum Publishing Corporation
233 Spring Street, New York, N.Y. 10013

Printed in the United States of America

Foreword

The cholesterol campaign has come to children. Just like the smoking campaign that started in the 1960s and the blood pressure campaign that started in the 1970s, when every child (and every adult, too) had to find out his or her blood pressure numbers. If those numbers are elevated, they must be controlled in childhood. Now, we want children to find out their cholesterol level.

Not quite half the children in North America, in most industrialized countries, and even in the large cities of the third world will die of what we call the *atherosclerotic diseases*; other terms are *heart attack*, *stroke*, and *peripheral vascular disease*. One-third of us experience a clinical event before the age of sixty-five. These diseases begin in childhood, usually in the large artery in our abdomen; they begin as deposits of cholesterol, bright yellow spots dotting the surface of this large artery. These *fatty streaks*, as we call them, spread in two ways. Locally, they start to get thicker. Some of the thickness is due to a type of scar tissue called *connective tissue*, as well as to the swollen cells full of cholesterol deposits. They also spread to other arteries: They go to the heart arteries, then to the big artery in the chest, then into the legs, into the neck, and finally into the brain. In Framingham, we have been looking inside the arteries of the neck—that is, the carotid arteries—with ultrasound, a procedure that is noninvasive and takes only twenty minutes to perform. Using sound that bounces back, we get a picture that is a little bit like a radar picture, but without any toxicity. Of the men and women of Framingham, 76 percent have cholesterol deposits large enough so that they can be seen easily by ultrasound. Of all the men and women in Framingham, 10 percent have a 50 percent blockage or worse. As mentioned above, once cholesterol deposits are in the neck, they are also in heart arteries, and they began to build up in childhood.

Our national councils, formed by the National Heart, Lung, and Blood Institute, part of our National Institutes of Health, have drawn up new guidelines for finding those persons who are destined to have a heart attack because their cholesterol levels are too high. The Framingham Heart Study was one of the earliest studies to show that the higher the cholesterol level, the higher the chance of a heart attack. Since then, studies from all over the world have shown that, if you lower your cholesterol level, you can prevent a heart attack. Now the Report of the Expert Panel on Blood Cholesterol Levels in Children and Adolescents has given us the dangerous numbers for children.

If your child has a total cholesterol level over 170 milligrams per deciliter, she or he is no longer "normal" and needs to be doing something constructive about lowering this cholesterol level. At least 25 percent of all children have a level over this number, and some studies show 30 percent are there. Many children have cholesterol levels over 200. These children, we fear, have a head start on this terrible epidemic, which kills twice as many people in our country as all the cancers put together.

What can you do in the face of all this? Where can you find out what the cholesterol numbers mean? What should children do? Do they need to take drugs? Are all the fast-food places equally bad? This book provides the practical answers to all

these questions by a doctor who has spent his professional life
answering them. It gives simple, straightforward answers that
are easy to understand and practical enough so all parents can
start to help their children take a different road in life—a road
with a better diet and exercise, and with an attitude that
protects health and prevents the awful consequences of our too-
rich lifestyle and slovenly habits. Genes count and family
history counts. To add up *all* the things that count, you need a
solid place to turn to for good advice. This book is a great place
to start.

WILLIAM P. CASTELLI, M.D.

Director
Framingham Heart Study
National Heart, Lung, and Blood Institute

Acknowledgments

We want to thank everyone who helped us throughout the preparation of this book, especially the following:

William P. Castelli, M.D., Director of the Framingham Heart Study, and Marc S. Jacobson, M.D., Director of the Atherosclerosis Prevention Program of the Schneider Children's Hospital, for their encouragement.

Maura Curless for her creative contribution to two chapters and Lisa Greissinger for her accurate and thorough work in compiling the dietary tables and all those wonderful recipes.

Nancy Copperman, registered dietician, for demonstrating an effective and cheerful approach to her work with children and their families in the treatment of high cholesterol levels.

Vic Dante, Lesley Howe, and the Crosby Street Studios for their practical and fun approach to achieving physical fitness in children.

Jan Kirshner, public relations expert, for getting us together with Julian Bach, our wise and experienced literary agent, who saw merit in our work.

Ann Seraphine-Han for her energy in spreading the good word about our effort to combat high cholesterol levels in children.

Lee Schreiber, empathetic friend and author, who gave counsel and reassurance, and Ethel Stogol, a wise and experienced editor, who made numerous useful suggestions with her customary total honesty.

Roz Reiman and Donna Hanc, who brought our writing team together and gave unstinting support throughout the planning and preparation of this book.

Contents

Introduction

Every day, I look into the eyes of children.

I see dozens of children, from all backgrounds; of all ages, sizes, shapes, and colors; with varied intelligence levels, talents, and temperaments. In and out of my office they come, hands held by their concerned parents. Some are afraid to look me in the eye. Others gaze back at me, cool and confident as fighter pilots. All, in their own special way, are precious.

Although they usually have symptoms I can see, hear, smell, or somehow detect, I can't help but think that, lurking beneath the surface, like some great white shark about to attack, is one of the single greatest threats to their health. It is something I can't pick up with a stethoscope or even an X ray. It's a silent threat and, make no mistake about it, a deadly one.

Cholesterol.

Most people are aware of cholesterol's dangers. They know how it can gradually clog the arteries and literally choke off the heart from its blood supply. And yet, whereas an entire industry has developed to help adults who are trying to lower their cholesterol levels, there's hardly anything available for parents who want to do the same for their children.

Ironic, isn't it? Especially when you realize that the younger you are, the better the results of a healthier lifestyle can be. Indeed, this book was prompted by my own frustration as a

1

pediatrician by the irony and inequity of this situation. When parents wanted information about cholesterol and their children and asked what to do about it, I had little to give them outside of a few pamphlets. What I could give them was advice — advice that I would now like to share with you.

Much of the information in this book is based on four decades of research about cholesterol and children, conducted by scientists around the world. But the program itself — the "how" as opposed to the "why" — is not coming to you from a researcher. These are the words of a doctor, a doctor who sees children much like yours every day.

I've been a pediatrician for thirty-nine years. In the past eight years, since I started routine testing for cholesterol in all of my young patients, I've advised thousands of parents on how to reduce cholesterol levels in their kids — not just by reciting the technical aspects, but by offering methods that recognize the realities of parenting. That's why we've included chapters on such real-world issues as shopping with your children, what your children eat in school, and how to get them to comply with the program.

The good news is that cholesterol levels, which are high in a significant percentage of American children, can be reduced in most cases. The researchers have proved it in the labs. I've seen the proof in my office with my own patients. These families have done it, and so can you. They've successfully lowered their children's cholesterol levels (and often, I should add, their own), without making radical changes in their lives and without using dangerous or controversial methods. Rather, this program advocates common sense along with a judicious modification of diet and lifestyle.

I've never been comfortable with quick fixes or eight-week cures. Although this program will enable you to see results quickly, it's really an investment — one of the smartest you can make for your children's future. By getting them into the mindset of healthy and proper eating habits now, you'll be saving them from the misery of heart disease tomorrow. And believe me, no matter how great our advances in treating heart disease (and they have been tremendous), it will always be a lot easier to prevent than to treat later on.

Besides, my approach for lowering your kids' cholesterol levels is really quite easy to understand — and to live with. This program won't turn you into a joyless, miserable person. Nor will it make social outcasts out of your kids. Your own doctor will agree with it; she or he will recognize that it's a prescription for better living and a program that can help you, too.

Although our first goal is to reduce cholesterol levels, and our long-term goal is to prevent heart disease, the most gratifying and immediate benefit is the improvement that this program can make in your quality of life: the way you look, the way you feel, and the way you enjoy each day. To me, that's the best gift you can give to your children, and to yourself.

So take a good look into your child's eyes and let's get started.

1

Cholesterol
The Silent Killer in Your Child

Back when I was a young medical student, we were taught that heart disease was simply part of growing old, and that part of the treatment was getting patients to accept their condition and live with it as best they could.

Now we know that the answer isn't acceptance; it's action, action that is best taken early in life. For most people, potential heart problems, in the form of high cholesterol levels, begin in childhood and therefore can be prevented in childhood.

Cholesterol. There's that nasty word we've all been hearing so much about. The way it's bandied about in the media, you'd think it was a toxic substance or some kind of unnatural poison. In truth, nothing could be more natural than cholesterol. Look it up in the dictionary and you'll find a definition like this: "A fatty substance present in animal cells and body fluids, important in physiological processes."

Indeed, cholesterol is important: in the formation of the cell membranes that protect your nervous system; in the manufacture of hormones, such as estrogen and progesterone; and in the digestive process. A little cholesterol is actually a good

5

thing. It's harmless looking, too, resembling nothing more threatening than melted candle wax.

And yet, this substance that is so essential to life that it is manufactured by our own bodies has been proved to be a primary cause of the number one killer in America: heart disease.

Very simply, it works this way: When there is too much cholesterol in the bloodstream, it begins to collect in the walls of the coronary arteries. These arteries, which are vital in supplying blood to the heart, start to lose their elasticity and their ability to regulate blood flow and pressure. Eventually, the arteries get so clogged by the cholesterol that they become completely blocked.

We'll talk a little more about the different types of cholesterol and how they're produced, measured, and controlled later in this chapter. Don't worry, this isn't a science textbook, and you're not going to be quizzed. But I do think it's important that you understand something about cholesterol before we can get down to the business of reducing it in your child.

I say *understand*, not *misunderstand*. I realize you've already heard a great deal about cholesterol — maybe too much, in fact. But almost all of what you've heard has pertained to adults. There's been almost nothing in the popular press about the effects of cholesterol on young people — effects that, I want to emphasize, are well documented by over forty years of worldwide studies.

What all of the research points to is this: The high levels of cholesterol that are proved to cause atherosclerosis — the "hardening" of the arteries we mentioned before — starts in childhood. In other words, the heart disease time bomb is ticking right now in millions of children, in America, Europe, Japan, and anywhere else that enjoys our kind of "Western" lifestyle. In rural China, by comparison, the people may have problems, but high cholesterol certainly isn't one of them. The average Chinese child has one-third less cholesterol than his American counterpart.

So while it's fine for adults to reduce their cholesterol — and I urge you to do so, along with your child — it's even more important to start young.

Remember the height charts your parents used to paste up on your bedroom wall when you were a kid? You would write down what height you were at a certain age and keep track of your progress as you grew, thinking — if you were like my kids — that maybe someday you'd hit the ceiling. The cholesterol "height chart" isn't as much fun, but it does illustrate a sad fact of life in our modern society — a fact, I hasten to say again, that can be changed.

Researchers have found what they call *fatty infiltrates* in the aorta — the main artery of the body — in children as young as three. Yes, three years old. Although I try not to use medical jargon with parents, that term *fatty infiltrates* is so chillingly descriptive that I want to emphasize it. What it says, graph-ically, is that dangerous amounts of fat, far more than the body needs, have infiltrated those perfect, beautiful bodies almost as soon as your children have learned to walk and talk. While some of these high fat levels are found in children who are genetically predisposed toward high cholesterol levels, the majority of them are not. These kids have high cholesterol levels because of what they've been fed. That's not only dangerous, in my view, it's a national disgrace.

By the ages of ten to twelve, we see that the problem has grown worse. Thick, fibrous lesions, less reversible than the early deposits, are beginning to develop. These deep bands of fat have grown to the point where they're now protruding into the passageways of the arteries themselves. What we see here, in elementary-school-aged children, is the beginning of a tragic

.

process that could end with a coronary bypass — the procedure that's performed when those arteries are so blocked by fat that blood can't even flow.

Finally, by the time our youngsters are old enough to vote, when they're vigorous, vital, and at the peak of their physical prowess, many of them already have the hearts of middle-aged men. How do we know this? From studies that were done on casualties in the Korean and Vietnam wars. Many of these brave young soldiers — a generation apart — had tired, old hearts, marbled with fat, primed for heart disease. Had they survived the fighting, many of these men (average age, 22) would have been battling for their lives in a coronary care unit in the not-too-distant future.

It's a sad and shocking story. Yet, I think it can have a happy ending, at least for many of the families that I see in my practice. I think these children will have a good chance to write a different story for their lives, a story that won't end someday in a cardiac care unit, because their parents are following the same simple, commonsense principles that I'm going to share with you.

But first, let's take a closer look at the silent killer — and people's understanding and misunderstanding of it. I will start with a case from my own practice.

I had just finished examining Susie, a thin, pretty three-year old, and everything seemed just fine. "Now," I told her mother, "we'll take a drop of blood from her finger for a blood count, and at the same time, we'll check her cholesterol level. I'll have the result for you in just a few minutes." Susie had no family history of heart disease except for one grandfather, who had died of a heart attack.

Three minutes later, I was back with the report. Susie's cholesterol level was 235. We'll talk about interpreting these numbers in the next chapter, but I can tell you now that that's very high. I discussed the results with Susie's mom, a petite ex-schoolteacher. I tried to make the point that, although it was a high reading, there was no immediate risk to Susie. We had our work cut out for us, certainly, but there was no reason to panic or to label Susie "sick."

At that moment, Susie's mom began to cry. "I'm having trouble accepting this," she said between sobs. "One day I read that we should check young children for their cholesterol level, and the next day, I read that there's inadequate evidence for doing it. And now you're telling me there's a problem. I don't know what to believe."

I sympathized with her. If you take your information from the churning sea of conflicting studies and opinions that flow through the pages of your newspaper and on TV talk shows, the issue of cholesterol and your child is a frustrating and confusing one. However, in my office that day, I gently explained to Susie's mom that the test was a warning sign — not a death warrant or even a hospital admission ticket — and that what we had to do now was heed that warning. Unlike some of the childhood diseases I've seen and had to share with parents, a high cholesterol count is something that *can* be corrected. This explanation helped Susie's mom. Now, she was ready to deal with the problem.

THE PROBLEM

This young mother's problem was with her child's high cholesterol level. Our society's problem with cholesterol among both children and adults is much greater in scope, and yet, so many people — even a few that should know better — seem to want to ignore or minimize this problem, thinking that if they do so, it will just go away like a headache. It's even become fashionable lately to say that the whole cholesterol issue has become overblown, and that we're putting too much emphasis on it as opposed to other aspects of health.

One of the naysayers is Russell Baker, who is not a physician, but an insightful and usually delightful writer. "Cholesterol shmolesterol," he wrote in the *New York Times* of November 29, 1989. "If you cannot do anything better than feel good about your cholesterol, you are close to life's bottom." He went on to extol the virtues of the "good" old-fashioned breakfast of bacon, eggs, buttered toast, milk, and coffee. See the analysis of this breakfast in Table 1.

Many would accuse us of sabotaging childhood itself. What cruel and inhuman punishment it is to deny red-blooded American children their cheeseburgers, french fries, and milkshakes or to take the ice cream cones right out of their mouths! Maybe, these people say, it's important for people of Russell Baker's age to watch their diet, but would you really deprive a child of these treats?

I wouldn't dream of it—as long as such high-fat foods are served in moderation or alternatives are substituted that are similar but lower in fat. Besides, that argument obscures the dimensions of the real problems. Here, the facts speak far too loudly—even louder than the voices of the naysayers and the fence sitters. Let's consider a few of them:

- Every thirty-two seconds, someone in this country dies of heart disease.
- Coronary heart disease causes more deaths than all forms of cancer combined.
- One out of every two men, women, and children in the United States will eventually succumb to heart attack or stroke.
- In the United States, 5.4 million people are known to have symptoms of heart disease, 1.5 million will actually

Table 1. The Russell Baker Good "Old-Fashioned" Breakfast (Analysis)

Food	Calories	Grams of fat (%)	Grams of saturated fat (%)	Milligrams of cholesterol
Bacon, 2 slices	73	6.2 gm. (76.4%) (55.8 calories)	2.2 gm. (27.1%) (19.8 calories)	11
2 eggs, fried in butter	188	14.4 gm. (68.9%) (129.6 calories)	5.4 gm. (26.0%) (48.6 calories)	558
White bread, 2 slices	140	2.0 gm. (12.8%) (18 calories)	1.0 gm. (6.4%) (9 calories)	2
Butter, 1 tbs.	103	11.4 gm. (100%) (102 calories)	7.1 gm. (62.6%) (63.9 calories)	31
Whole milk, 1 cup	150	8.2 gm. (49.2%) (73.8 calories)	5.1 gm. (30.6%) (45.9 calories)	33
Coffee, 1 cup	0	0	0	0
Cream, 1 tbs.	29	2.9 gm. (86.2%) (25 calories)	1.8 gm. (55.8%) (16.2 calories)	10
Total	682	45.1 gm. (59.5%) (405.9 calories)	22.6 gm. (29.9%) (203.4 calories)	645

have a heart attack, and one-third of these attacks will
be fatal.
- The direct and indirect costs of heart disease add up to
more than $50 billion annually — money that could have
gone to build new schools, clean up our rivers, or help
find a cure for muscular dystrophy.

Sobering statistics, indeed. But think for a minute: What
do all of these people have in common? An exhaustive review of
the evidence leads to an inescapable conclusion: Whether they
knew it or not (and they probably didn't), most of the people
who have had or who will have heart disease had high cholesterol levels in childhood. Yes, the heart disease that has dam-
aged and, in many cases, snuffed out these lives had its roots
in childhood. The higher the cholesterol level of a child, the
greater the likelihood of coronary heart disease in the adult.
Reducing the level, therefore, reduces the risk.

It's really that simple, and at this point, the evidence is
unassailable. There is no longer any controversy about the role
of cholesterol in heart disease. It has been established beyond
any reasonable doubt that an elevated blood cholesterol level is
a major cause of coronary artery disease. It has also been
established — through test after test, study after study, year
after year — that lowering the level of cholesterol reduces that
risk. How can we lower our cholesterol levels? Primarily through
diet; secondarily, through exercise and other lifestyle modifications; finally, and in only the most extreme cases, through
drugs.

I don't want to mislead you here. High cholesterol is not the
only cause of heart disease. You're probably familiar with some
of the other "risk factors," such as smoking, high blood pressure, obesity, physical inactivity, and diabetes. Risk is also
affected by age, sex, and family history (as I suspect was little

Susie's case). You'll notice a similarity in most of these under-lying causes of heart disease. This is not an illness caused by viruses or bacteria. It's a disease caused by a way of life — a way of life found in rich, "developed," Western nations like ours. Comparisons of different populations throughout the world show a direct correlation between cholesterol levels and coronary heart disease: The higher the cholesterol level, the higher the frequency of heart disease. When economic conditions and lifestyles in countries have "improved" — such as in Japan and Korea — the average cholesterol levels have gone up and, with them, the number of heart attacks. Interestingly enough, the reverse is true, as well. Studies have shown that, when people from these countries move to other, less developed nations, their cholesterol levels and their risk of heart attacks drop.

Given this evidence, some might be tempted to call heart disease the price we pay for being a developed nation — a penalty of wealth, if you will, just like high taxes and too many cable channels. Although there may be some truth in view, it doesn't mean that we have to return to being an agrarian society in order to defeat this silent killer. It's not a matter of rewinding progress; it's a question of revising or at least refining our lifestyles, our diets, and our health practices, which we have already started to do. Witness the dramatic reduction in smok-ing and the increase, at least among certain segments of the population, in exercise and fitness awareness.

So why is it that, in approximately the time it took you to read that paragraph about how Americans are taking steps to minimize some factors that cause heart disease, about two more Americans died of heart disease? I'm not a sociologist, but I suspect that one reason is the false feeling of security among some people, the feeling that no matter what they do to break or damage their bodies, medical science will somehow have a pill or a procedure to fix it.

The truth is that we do have many ways to deal with heart disease once it's happened. In the past, physicians treating advanced cases of coronary artery disease could do little more than watch and wait for the inevitable. Today, watchful waiting is no longer our most practiced art form. We live in an age of active intervention in medicine: drugs, angioplasty, or open-heart bypass surgery. These are all marvelous lifesaving methods. They're also very complex and expensive procedures.

Many health-care practitioners, including this one, favor a different approach to dealing with heart disease: a preventive approach. Recently, a panel of thirty-eight health organizations, ranging from the American Heart Association to the American Medical Association, united in urging Americans to reduce their fat consumption to no more than 30 percent of their daily calories (and there's talk now of lowering that percentage).

Why such a rare display of unanimity? Because the members of these groups know that lowering your fat intake is likely to lower your cholesterol level. In fact, it's estimated that diet alone can reduce total cholesterol by an average of 10 to 15 percent, and every 1 percent reduction in cholesterol is associated with at least a 2 percent reduction in coronary risk.

Those are encouraging numbers, but what discourages me is that almost all of the emphasis is being placed on prevention among adults. I deal with children, and I see their alarmingly high cholesterol levels, and their increasing obesity levels. The sad truth is that, although their parents are out jogging or taking aerobic classes, American kids are getting fatter, and in doing so, they're increasing their risk of heart disease. Experts estimate that two in five children between the ages of six and seventeen are overweight. And up to 30 percent of children — even those who aren't obese — have cholesterol levels over 170. To see how dangerous that is, let's take a closer look at the silent killer.

THE SILENT KILLER:
WHEN IT STARTS AND HOW IT WORKS

A major cause of heart disease is a condition called *athero-sclerosis*. This occurs when fat accumulates in the linings of the arteries, including the coronary arteries, those all-important pathways through which the blood transports oxygen and nutrients to the heart. If untreated, the arteries get so blocked up (occluded) with fat that blood can't get through to feed the heart.

Like the words *high cholesterol level* and *coronary heart disease*, *atherosclerosis* usually conjures up images of older adults, suffering from heart attacks brought on by decades of smoking or drinking or eating too many "good old-fashioned" breakfasts. The *last* thing associated with atherosclerosis is energetic children. Yet, in many cases, it's in childhood that this disease really begins.

The earliest signs of atherosclerosis are those fatty streaks I mentioned earlier, which are often present by the age of three. The numbers of these streaks of fat — which you can visualize as the marbled fat you see in raw meat — increase with age. Their buildup can be stopped and even reversed. All too often, however, those streaks go on to become thick, fibrous plaques — a sort of arterial garbage dump composed not only of fat, but of scar tissue, blood, and other unappetizing things.

The plaques are first seen during the preadolescent years. As they grow, they begin to protrude into the artery itself. Seventy-seven percent of the young American soldiers killed in Korea and 45 percent of those killed in Vietnam were found to have these plaques in their coronary arteries.

In autopsies of children who died from other causes, fatty lesions were found in the aorta and, to some extent, in the

coronary arteries. These children had no symptoms of atherosclerosis, such as the chest pains and shortness of breath that
will hurry an adult to his or her cardiologist. Because of this
absence of any such symptoms or signs of problems among
children, we call cholesterol a silent killer. However, make
no mistake about it; although it would take many years for
symptoms to develop, they were well on their way. Only one
clue suggested the problems to come, a clue that the researchers
doing these postmortem examinations discovered. There was
an "amazing relationship" between how high the blood cholesterol levels were and the extent of these fatty deposits in the
arteries. The process would progress gradually, but it would
only be when blockage exceeded tolerable limits that the
symptoms would surface.

Had these young people survived, chances are strong that
their fibrous plaques would have grown to the point of blocking
up almost an entire artery. That's when strokes and coronary
artery disease occur, and by then, preventive measures are often
too little, too late.

The key lesson to be learned from these and many other
ongoing studies is that elevated cholesterol levels begin in
childhood. The direct correlation between high cholesterol —
that odorless, colorless, waxy substance produced naturally
by the body and supplemented through diet — and the number
and extent of the fatty streaks and fibrous plaques that appear
in the arteries of children cannot be disputed. The unfortunate
results will first be seen by physicians other than pediatricians,
who will care for our child patients after they have grown into
adults.

How does this process occur? Indeed, how does cholesterol
do its not-always-dirty work? To understand how to prevent high
cholesterol levels, it's important to understand a little bit about
how cholesterol works and, indeed, what it really is.

Cholesterol is a waxy substance produced by the body that, when combined, with proteins, is called *lipoprotein*. Where does the *lipo* come in? It refers to fats or "lipids," and even though cholesterol is not technically a fat, the term has come into common usage, even in the scientific community, perhaps because excessive cholesterol in the body is a result of excessive fat in the diet.

The term *total cholesterol* (which is the number you'll see when your child is tested) really refers to the sum total of the different types of lipoproteins found in the blood; each of them contains cholesterol, as well as various and specific kinds of protein. What is of utmost importance to your child's health is which of these different types of lipoproteins are present, and in what percentages. In fact, I often think that what we should be asking is not "What's your cholesterol level?" but "What's your lipoprotein level?" "Which ones do you have?" and "How much?"

I could go on for pages and pages trying to explain the chemical and molecular combination of the various cholesterols. Indeed, tomes have been written about such topics, mostly of interest to the inner medical research fraternity. While not diminishing the importance of such work (it is, after all, the foundation of our knowledge), I'll let you in on a secret: for most pediatricians, such scientific arcana are not relevant to our diagnosis or treatment of cholesterol problems in our patients. So I'll spare you, as well. I think that what's most important for a parent to understand is that there are different forms of cholesterol-carrying lipoproteins, and that some are good and some are not so good. Let's run them down:

First, let's get back to this term *lipoprotein*. *Lipo*, as we said, refers to fat. But how did protein get into the act? When cholesterol is introduced into the body, it combines with proteins. This combination is what makes cholesterol soluble, so that it can flow in the blood. Otherwise, it would be a non-soluble waxy lump floating through the bloodstream like an iceberg in a remote ocean — a mere curiosity, as it was in the eighteenth and early nineteenth centuries, when cholesterol (which hadn't even been named yet) was known only as a major component of gallstones.

We've learned in the years since that cholesterol is a more complex substance. It combines with different types of proteins into three combinations of lipoproteins, the sum of which we measure as "total cholesterol":

- *Low-density lipoprotein* (LDL) carries the cholesterol to the cells (which is good) and also deposits *excess* cholesterol on the linings of the arteries (which is not so good).
- *Very-low-density lipoprotein* (VLDL) makes up the smallest percentage among the various major combinations of cholesterol and protein. VLDL performs a similarly unsavory role after being converted into LDL.
- *High-density lipoprotein* (HDL) works to *remove* cholesterol from the arterial walls and brings it back to the liver for elimination from the body.

There's nothing sinister or unnatural about this balancing act. LDL and VLDL are not accumulated by eating too many eggs or watching the wrong TV shows. Indeed, we can visualize it as one of the body's ongoing balancing acts. What we're aiming for in this program is to maintain that balance, which is thrown off when we have too much LDL (the lipoprotein that leaves cholesterol behind on the walls of the arteries) and not enough HDL to scrub it off. It's then that the slow, decades-long buildup starts, from streaks to plaques to hospital bed.

But let's not forget that some cholesterol is necessary, especially during the first two years of life. This is why we never test cholesterol levels or recommend any fat restrictions in the diets of children under two years of age. Beyond that age, it's a different story. Once the nervous system is formed, the brain is more fully developed, and the sheer velocity of the body's growth (most of which occurs in those first two years of life) begins to slow down, we have to be careful. That's when children begin to build up cholesterol levels, often into alarming numbers.

In the United States alone, at least one-third of all the children aged two to eighteen have higher cholesterol levels than they should (over 170), so that they have a moderate potential risk of future heart disease. And about 10 percent have cholesterol levels that are very high (over 200) and that — if left untreated — will put them on the road to becoming one of the statistics I cited earlier.

It doesn't have to be that way: We can take precautionary steps. The question is when. Progress has already been made, as the difference in the degree of coronary artery disease between casualties from the Korean War and Vietnam — about fifteen years later — attests. Most of that improvement can be attributed to a reduction in smoking and an increase in exercise among the troops of the two different eras. But now, we have an opportunity to accelerate this process even more, with a sensible diet, as well as other lifestyle changes.

Once, after we had been discussing this very topic, one of my mothers threw up her hands.

"Dr. Reiman," she said impatiently, "my child is five years old. She's only a kid. She's healthy and energetic. Why do we have to torture ourselves? Can't we worry about heart disease when she's older?"

The answer, in a word, is "no." Because, as you've seen, the problem will only be worse then. Don't we owe it to our children to put them on the right path, the path that will help them avoid the nightmare of heart disease? And besides, as

you'll see in the coming chapters, the diet and lifestyle modifications we're suggesting are hardly torturous. If anything,
they'll take your beautiful, energetic young children and make
them even more so — adding to the quality of their lives, and
yours.

Let's start preventing heart disease right now. Let's do it
as a family, and let's begin by having your children tested — and
you and your spouse, as well, if you haven't been tested already!

2

Cholesterol Tests
Why We Do Them, How We Do Them, and What They Mean

The following three proven facts lead us to one powerful conclusion:

Fact 1: Atherosclerotic disease is the number one killer of adults in the industrial world.

Fact 2: Reducing risk factors in adults reduces the risk of this disease.

Fact 3: Atherosclerosis begins in childhood.

It adds up to this: If we start modifying risk factors early in childhood, the silent killer can be silenced. We can minimize atherosclerosis, slow its progress, or prevent it altogether.

How do we determine the extent to which your child may be at risk? By testing. (And remember, please, it's not an immediate but a long-term risk we're talking about.)

In school, your child takes tests to see how well he or she can write, add, or subtract. The results help teachers determine whether your child has potential problems in those areas. In the pediatrician's office, we do the same thing to determine whether your child has a potential cholesterol problem.

The question of which children to test is one of the most divisive issues in pediatrics today. There are some, as you will see, who advocate testing only those children with a family history of early heart problems (defined as having one or more parents or grandparents who died of heart disease at less than fifty years of age). But it's been estimated that if we tested only those children, we would still miss a full 50 percent of those who are at risk. Many children with no family history of heart disease may nevertheless face a risky future if they and their parents don't begin to take steps now.

WHY WE TEST

Cholesterol screening is the third most commonly recommended medical test in adults, after blood pressure measurement and Pap smears. It is *the* most common blood measurement.

Yet, as late as 1988, only 14 percent of pediatricians and 8 percent of family physicians were doing "universal" cholesterol screenings, that is, routine screening among all of their young patients. Seventy-seven percent of the pediatricians and about 70 percent of all family doctors measured children with family histories of cardiovascular disease.

My associates and I were among those 14 percent. We've being doing universal screening of our children since 1985. We felt a bit like the odd men out back then, but we sensed that this was the right approach. The increasing numbers of pediatricians who are opting for universal screening (we suspect it's now up to between one-third and one-half) are helping to affirm that decision. Still, there is resistance. Let's take a look at why some in the medical community continue to oppose universal screening.

UNIVERSAL TESTING: THE CASE AGAINST IT

Those against universal screening aren't against *any* cholesterol testing among children. They just feel it's best to screen only if one of the following conditions exist:

1. A parent has a blood cholesterol level over 240.
2. A parent or a grandparent had a heart attack* at or before age fifty.
3. A parent or a grandparent had atherosclerosis at or before age fifty.

Although many of those in favor of targeted screening agree that atherosclerosis begins in childhood and is related to cholesterol levels in childhood, they still favor this limited testing. Their reasons:

1. Many children who have high childhood levels have almost normal levels when they become adults.
2. Widespread testing may result in many children being labeled as having a disease that may never occur.
3. We may cause needless anxiety.
4. Universal testing may lead to the overuse of cholesterol-lowering drugs.

I don't want to disparage the views of my well-meaning colleagues, which is why I presented them to you first without

*We've already defined atherosclerosis as the gradual closing down of an artery. When one of the major coronary arteries becomes totally closed off by plaque, the part of the heart muscle that is nourished by that artery will die. The death of that portion of heart muscle is a myocardial infarction, or a heart attack.

comment, but before I go on to explain the case for universal screening, and why I think you should test your children regardless of family history, I would now like to rebut a few of these objections, which received wide publicity when they were released as part of the 1991 National Cholesterol Education Project's recommendations:

1. *"Many children who have high childhood levels have almost normal levels when they become adults."* Well, what of the many who don't? And how many of them don't because they woke up to diet and lifestyle changes — the same ones that could have been made in childhood — as adults, maybe just in the nick of time? By the same token, should we encourage teenage smokers to wait and quit only after they develop a hacking cough? This strikes me as a twist on the kind of thinking behind the federal budget deficit. Let somebody else worry about it tomorrow.

2. *"Widespread testing could result in children's being labeled as having a disease."* Pure semantics. If your financial adviser tells you that you'd better start saving for your child's college education now, does that mean you are suddenly faced with a financial crisis? You will be if you wait fifteen years to do something about it, maybe, but not this minute. It's the same thing with awareness of cholesterol levels. What if we called it an *opportunity* instead, an opportunity for parents to help their children learn to follow sensible eating habits and maintain a healthier lifestyle? Or a wake-up call, to plan ahead? I find this rush to "protect" parents — as if they were the children — offensive.

3. *"We may cause needless anxiety."* Why must we assume that health professionals are so inept at counseling, or that parents are so neurotic, that we must somehow shield them from legitimate medical information that they are entitled to? Indeed, most of the mothers and fathers I deal with are already informed and eager for *more* information about every aspect of parenting — not *less*.

4. *"Universal testing may lead to the overuse of drugs."* At present, only 1 percent of children, those with stubbornly and perilously high cholesterol levels, are treated with cholesterol-lowering drugs such as colestipol or cholestyramine, and only 7 percent of pediatricians have ever prescribed such drugs even once in their careers.

UNIVERSAL TESTING: THE CASE FOR IT

Let's look at this question from a broader perspective. Is it truly worthwhile to screen an entire population of children to identify the percentage who will benefit from intervention for *any* disease or potential problem? We now screen newborns for phenylketonuria (a metabolic disease that causes mental retardation) when the proportion who have it is 1 in 14,000. And we universally screen for congenital hypothyroidism when its incidence is 1 in 4,000.

Cardiovascular disease, on the other hand, is the most common health disorder in the country and the leading killer of adults. So how do we justify not screening for high cholesterol levels, the most reliable early predictor of that disease?

When I debate this question with the steadily dwindling number of my colleagues who oppose universal screening, I answer their question "Why?" with "Why not?" Why *not* screen all children? Considering the early appearance of plaques in the coronary arteries and the proven effectiveness of screening, education, and treatment programs among adults, there is all the more reason to initiate the same procedures for children. After all, it's a lot easier to change eating and behavioral habits in the young.

Besides, if we test only those with a family history of heart disease, we'll miss half the children who may be at risk because of high cholesterol. In one study of 6,000 children screened for total cholesterol levels, 10 to 15 percent were over 200 and 1 percent over 250. Of these, 40 percent would have been missed if only the "at-risk" group had been tested. Other studies have shown that 48 percent of children with LDL levels as high as the 95th percentile had no family history of heart disease.

To a pediatrician, the possibility of missing all those children—who could easily have been helped—is absolutely unacceptable. That's why I urge you to have your child tested, whether or not you have a family history of heart problems. There are also other reasons not to limit screening just to those with family histories:

1. Family histories, sad to say, are becoming more and more difficult to reconstruct. Many of my children come from single-parent families, or from families in which the father is not the natural father. With increasing numbers of adoptions and with nearly half of all American marriages ending in divorce, medical information about natural parents and ex-spouses, not to mention ex-spouses' parents, gets sketchier and more fragmented.

2. Taking a good family history, even from intact families, may take twenty to thirty minutes. Most pediatricians don't do it, and even fewer update the information.

3. Most parents of young children are too young to show signs of coronary heart disease. I once attended a medical seminar in which the speaker, a physician herself, pointed out that, when her father had his first heart attack at age forty-nine, she was twenty-five years old and thus would have been missed in a childhood screening of only those with a positive family history. Needless to say, she now recommends universal screening.

4. In screening only children with a family history of heart disease, up to two-thirds of children at high risk may be missed.

On the other hand, 50 percent of children who do have such a family history have normal cholesterol levels. Obviously, the results are not predictable without the evidence of a cholesterol test.

5. We're not talking about an expensive or painful procedure here. The test of cholesterol levels is one of the fastest, easiest, most accurate, and least expensive tests a doctor can do. Certainly, it is far easier and less traumatic than the more than 260,000 coronary bypass operations done every year in the United States.

HOW WE DO THE CHOLESTEROL TEST

We recommend testing all children over the age of two, for two reasons. First, under the age of two, fat restriction is not recommended. It's during that explosive period of growth that fat is needed, so there's no point in measuring it. Second, the cholesterol level starts very low at birth — at an average of 70 — and reaches near-adult levels by the end of the second year. In fact, cholesterol levels go up only another 40 to 60 points, on average, during the rest of life.

The younger we start, the easier it is to change and modify diet and lifestyle, if such modifications are necessary. And, of course, as we discussed earlier, the first traces of heart disease — the fatty streaks in the arteries — can be detected as early as age three years. The longer cholesterol levels remain high, and the more they build up, the more difficult it may be to reverse the process. Those later fibrous plaques are even more difficult to get rid of than the initial fatty streaks. So if the idea is prevention, let's start preventing sooner rather than later.

How is cholesterol level measured? Until about 1985, cholesterol testing involved drawing blood from a vein, in a laboratory. Now, thanks to advances in medical technology, the test is much easier for me, for you, and for your child. We perform most of our tests right in the office. A single drop of blood is all that's needed, and when the test is done properly, we get amazingly accurate results. The margin of error of our cholesterol-testing machines is, at most, 3 percent and is getting lower all the time.

"Done properly" means that the machines are calibrated in our office every morning and again after every twenty tests. In addition, a duplicate specimen should be routinely sent to a reliable outside lab so that the results can be compared for control purposes.

As I said, we've had our machine since it became available on the market in 1985. We use a Reflotron, made by Boehringer-Mannheim, which is one of the most commonly used types of machine. Kodak and Abbott laboratories also manufacture machines. A pediatrician who doesn't have the capability to do the test in his or her own office is not necessarily underestimating the dangers of cholesterol. The testing equipment can be prohibitively expensive. Instead, ask him or her to refer you to a reliable local lab.

I don't recommend that you get your child's cholesterol tested at a shopping mall or in other public places where mass testing is done. Although I appreciate the role these public screenings have played in raising awareness about cholesterol levels, we want to be sure that the results are accurate — and we often can't be sure in those situations.

THE TEST: WHAT TO EXPECT
AND HOW TO PREPARE

Your child's test should be done during what we call a "well visit," that is, during a regular checkup. Don't have your child tested when you've brought her or him in for an earache or a cold.

Your child does not have to fast before a cholesterol test, nor do you have to worry if she or he ate three pieces of birthday cake the day before. The test reflects all of the previous four to six weeks of diet.

I know this from a study I did on my own patients. In response to numerous questions from parents wondering whether high test scores could have been the result of weekend partying, I myself tracked a week of scores, from Monday through Friday. A total of 500 tests showed no Monday "weekend hangover" effect. The range of scores stayed the same each day through the week.

It may sound strange, but you should make sure of your child's physical position during the test. We have all of our children sit during the test. Other doctors may have them lie down. It doesn't matter which. What does matter is that, if you have to repeat the test, you should have it done the same way. Why? No one's sure of the reason, but total cholesterol levels tend to be a little lower when taken from patients who are lying down than when taken from those who are sitting up.

Finally, most pediatricians are gentle people, but we have to obtain a good and free flow of blood from the finger. If we're too gentle, the blood has to be "milked" — or squeezed — from the finger, and we get serum as well as whole blood. The result may be a sample that gives a false low reading of your child's cholesterol level.

The blood for most children's cholesterol tests is drawn by the "fingerstick" method, that is, pricking the fingertip with a small, sterile, disposable pin and then drawing the blood up through a thin plastic tube called a *pipette*. The blood is then pushed out onto a small magnetic tape, which is inserted into the cholesterol-testing machine. The machine shines a light through the blood and analyzes the composition of the sample electronically. In two-and-a-half minutes, the results flash on the screen.

Not only are they fast, cholesterol tests are less expensive than many of the medicines I prescribe. The average charge to the patient — including everything from the original cost of the equipment, office overhead, materials, interpretation, and counseling — is about twenty dollars. That's a real bargain for something that can change the course of your child's life, for the better. This is especially true when the cost is compared to that of a bypass operation, which may be awfully expensive by the year 2040, about the time when any of today's children are likely to need one.

INTERPRETING THE RESULTS

The blood is drawn without much trauma. We've already stuck a "Hero" sticker on our children's shirts before they realize what's happened. Your doctor disappears with the blood sample, returning a few minutes later to announce, "The cholesterol level is fine."

Ask the doctor for the number. The normal upper level for a child is 170 milligrams of cholesterol per 100 milliliters of blood (you'll often see the unit of measurement as "mg/100 ml"). The lower the number is, the better. There's no such thing as a cholesterol reading that's too low; in fact, our machine won't even bother showing a reading under 100. Remember, even though diet supplies about one-third of the cholesterol we use, the body is capable of producing all of the cholesterol we need. It's the excess cholesterol — which comes, in most cases, solely from diet — that we have to be concerned about.

Another scenario: Your doctor returns, frowns, and says,

"Hmmm. I have to tell you that the cholesterol level is a little high, but we can do something about it." He or she is right. You can do something about it. But first you should ask, "What is a little high?"

Borderline high is a level between 170 and 199. In our experience, having done almost thirty-thousand tests over nearly seven years, we've found that between one-quarter and one-third of all our children have levels in this range. So rest assured, you're not alone in this situation. Nevertheless, it is a situation that should be addressed.

One last possibility. Your doctor comes back into the office, as I have with Susie's mom and many others, sits down, and says something like this: "The cholesterol is pretty high and we really have to do something about it." What the doctor means is that your child's cholesterol level is over 200. What she or he does not mean is that your child has heart disease or is in imminent danger of having heart disease. As you learned from reading Chapter 1, atherosclerosis develops gradually, over several decades. You have plenty of time to do what you have to do—but you have to start doing something. And the sooner the better. Again, you're not alone. We've found in our practice that almost 15 percent of all the children we test are in this high range. It's distressing, but it shouldn't be depressing because, as I've said before, unlike some other conditions I've had to tell parents about, you can do something about this one.

In the case of this last scenario, you should consider two things: If your child's level is high, or even moderately high, the test should be repeated in two or three months. Is there a likelihood of error? Not in the machine itself, but as in anything else in our bodies, normal fluctuations take place. One two-week period of eating may not be the same as another. The amount of activity before the test may also have had an affect, a point we'll touch on later.

Further, if the test result is high, it would be very wise for you and your spouse to have *your* cholesterol levels checked, too. Many times, we've had children who have tested high, and sure enough, their parents then tested high as well. What surprises me sometimes is how many parents have not had their cholesterol levels measured or, if they have, don't recall the results.

If you already know that your own cholesterol level is high (over 200 for an adult), you should tell your pediatrician *before* your child's test. As part of his or her information gathering, your doctor will want to know this, as well as your spouse's cholesterol level, the levels of your child's blood siblings, and any heart problems, especially early (under fifty years of age) heart problems, among the grandparents. If your doctor doesn't ask you, tell him or her and ask that this information be made a part of your child's health record.

A CLOSER LOOK AT THE NUMBERS

The numbers we've been referring to are total cholesterol figures, that is, a combination of the LDL, HDL, and VLDL we discussed in Chapter 1.

If the total cholesterol level is normal (170 or lower), you need go no further, except to make sure you have the level tested again in a year. If it remains normal, then you can repeat it every two or three years (feel free to ask your pediatrician to include this as part of the routine testing of your child). Again, the lower the cholesterol level the better. So I urge you to skip to our chapters on diet, exercise, and behavior modification, because there's always room for improvement.

If the cholesterol level is high, don't wait for the repeat test to start making the kinds of changes we discuss at the end of this chapter and throughout the rest of the book. If it remains high on the second test, after dietary changes have been made for three to six months, then it may be prudent to learn the high-density lipoprotein (HDL), low-density lipoprotein (LDL), and very-low-density lipoprotein (VLDL) makeup of the total cholesterol. You can do that either at an outside laboratory or at a lipid clinic. Your pediatrician can recommend one in your area.

Here, the makeup of the cholesterol will be analyzed, just as it is when an internist does a blood workup on an adult, using a sample taken from the vein, as opposed to the finger. For this type of test, the blood must be drawn after a twelve-hour fast.

The results of this second, more extensive test will give you your child's levels of LDL, HDL, and VLDL. The VLDL levels, we should note, are sometimes derived indirectly by measurement of the triglycerides, another kind of fat that the body produces from leftover sugar. The breakdown is shown in the formula in Table 2.

For all practical purposes, the numbers you should pay attention to are the LDL and the HDL. The LDL, you'll recall, is the "bad" cholesterol that deposits the fat in the arteries. The HDL is the good guy, the body's street sweeper, cleaning out those arteries. And as in all things pertaining to our

Table 2. Components of Total Cholesterol

$TC = LDS + HDL + \frac{1}{5}TG^a$

TC: total cholesterol
LDS (or *LDL-C*): low-density lipoprotein
HDL (or *HDL-C*): high-density lipoprotein
TG: triglyceride
VLDL: very-low-density lipoprotein

---

[a]The formula is accurate except in the rare case where the triglyceride level is over 400.

bodies, we have guidelines that suggest what numbers for each are good or bad. These guidelines are shown in Table 3.

The important thing to remember is that the lower the LDL, the better, and the higher the HDL, the better. It would be nice if a high count of HDL is what accounts for a high total cholesterol number in your child's test. Unfortunately, although there is evidence that this is true among adult endurance athletes, it's not usually the case among children; in fact, only about 5 percent get off with this good excuse. It should be noted then that in 95 percent of all children with a high total cholesterol level, it's due to high LDL, not high HDL.

The interpretation of triglyceride levels should be left to the experts at your lipid clinic. Except in rare instances, they're not something to worry about in children. High triglycerides are a predominantly adult problem, and especially an LDL–triglyceride ratio over 4.5.

Table 3. Cholesterol-Level Guidelines for Children

LDL
Desirable: Less than 100
Borderline high: 110–129
Very high: 130 and over

HDL
Desirable: Above 45
Borderline low: 35–45
Very low: Below 35

Total cholesterol
Desirable: 170 or less
Borderline high: 171–199
Very high: 200 and over

TESTING: HOW RELIABLE IS IT?

The mother of a patient of mine who had tested high raised a question that you may be asking yourself: "I've heard that even if my child has a high cholesterol level, he may be fine when he's grown," this mother said. "So, Dr. Reiman, *why* are we going through all this trouble?"

The answer is that, for over twenty years, researchers have been *tracking* children as they grow older, checking to see how predictable these cholesterol measurements are. In other words, do high cholesterol levels among children inevitably lead to heart disease among those same children, when they grow up?

Fair question. Unlike for "tracking" studies done on other populations and for other diseases, we don't have fifty years of experience to draw on; little thought was given to cholesterol and children before 1970. However, we have been able to follow kids who had high cholesterol in the early 1970s and who are now young adults. An important ongoing study, which is being conducted by a group headed by Dr. Gerald Berenson of Louisiana State University Medical Center, has shown us this:

Of the children who were at high risk (those with total cholesterol levels of 200 or over), 81 percent were in the upper 50th percentile of cholesterol levels by the time they had reached adulthood; 62 percent were in the upper 25 percent, and 43 percent were in the upper 10 percent.

That's the answer I gave to the mother. The existing evidence — and we're gathering more every day — tells us that the cholesterol test results your child gets today are predictive of whether he or she will be a likely candidate for heart disease

as an adult. So, if your child has tested over 200 and you choose
to do nothing about it, the odds are 4 out of 5 that your child will
end up having an increased risk of heart disease as an adult. And
even if your child's level is moderately high, there is a high
likelihood that it will remain high—unless you choose to do
something about it now.

Either way, it's a gamble, and I don't like the odds. Neither
do most of my parents, and they choose to act. Knowing *how*
to act is the focus of much of the rest of this book.

FOLLOW-UP TESTING

No responsible pediatrician is going to hand you the result
of your child's cholesterol test without any explanation. In
fact, as I see it, getting the number is just the beginning of
the process, because the test numbers are just guidelines.
Action must be taken now.

First of all, don't panic if the number is high. Although you
have to face the reality of the situation, it's not such a terrible
reality. I'll say it again: This doesn't mean your child has a
disease—or will have one anytime soon. On the other hand,
I've seen all too many parents try to deny the fact that their
children have cholesterol problems. They blame the numbers
on a binge the day before, or they cite people who have high
cholesterol levels and never had a heart attack. To them, I say
we have to go by the odds—and we need to try to change them
so that they are in our favor. Besides, whatever we're doing is
going to be healthful and helpful. Our "treatment" is neither
onerous, painful, nor even expensive.

At this point, we begin counseling. Here's how I do it.
"Knowing everything you already know about nutrition and

lifestyle," I say, "can you visualize already some things that could be changed to help us lower Veronica's cholesterol level?"

I ask this because I try to respect the intelligence of my patients, and I recognize that most of the changes that will be made have to be made at home and under the *parents'* supervision, not mine. So ask yourself these questions:

- Is your child eating a lot of dairy products, red meat, eggs, and sweets?
- Is your child spending more time playing Super Mario Brothers on the TV than stickball?
- Is your child having a lot of snacks, and if so, what kinds?
- What's your child eating at school or in day care?
- Where do you go and what do you eat when you go out to eat?
- How do you plan your supermarket shopping?
- What's going on at grandma's house?
- Is your child overweight?

If you go back to the table of contents, you'll see that almost every one of these questions is addressed in this book. Virtually every aspect of your child's life—diet, exercise, and behavior in school and other outside situations, as well as the behavior and habits of the rest of your family—influences his or her cholesterol level (which, in turn, will affect the quality of his or her life).

Your pediatrician will try to work these various issues out with you, but keep in mind that one of the reasons for this book is my own frustration at not being able to spend adequate counseling time with the parents of each of my patients. I'm not alone. A large university study found that pediatricians spend an average of only one to five minutes per visit on counseling.

It's not that pediatricians don't recognize the importance of spending time with patients and their families. It's just that we don't have the time to spend with each of you that we'd like.

For now, make sure that your pediatrician has all of the relevant information about your family history that you can gather — including, of course, your own cholesterol levels. Then, turn the page, and let's get started on lowering your child's cholesterol.

3

Trimming the Fat

Tasteful Ways to Reduce Your Child's Risk

You don't have to wait for the test results to start reading this chapter. It's our belief that all children, no matter how low their cholesterol readings, will benefit from a diet that's lower in fats.

A healthy diet, of course, is not the only way to reduce cholesterol levels. In later chapters, we'll be talking about exercise, for example, an often overlooked component of cholesterol level control. But what we're going to concentrate on here and in the next few chapters is the issue of food, glorious food.

We're going to help you put together a diet for a healthy heart. This diet isn't just something you can live with, but something you and your family can really enjoy. Nor is it highly restrictive; it won't make your children feel like outcasts. On the contrary, they can have their ice cream. They can have their fast food. They can have their snacks. To deny kids these foods, I've found, is often counterproductive. After all, no matter what your children's cholesterol readings, they are still children and therefore have some basic needs. Over the years, there have been enough myths and misstatements about these needs to fill several books. What we're recommending here is a combination of the old and the new. The old is the still useful notion that kids should eat a balanced diet that includes servings from the various food groups. The new approach is the so-called Step One diet of the American Heart Association.

In this diet, it's recommended that 50 to 60 percent of total calories come from carbohydrates; 10 to 20 percent as protein and 30 percent as fats. We'll focus on fat because when it comes to the silent killer, this is truly the heart of the matter.

Our society has a thing against looking fat. Thin is in, models get skinnier every year, and people spend billions of dollars trying to sweat, fast, or drink the pounds away. If we're so down on fat, I often wonder, how come we eat so much of the stuff? There are a couple of good reasons. First of all, some fat is essential for protecting the vital organs of the body, and it serves as an energy source. Second, it does help our food taste better. But the simple truth is that too much fat, which is what the vast majority of American kids are being fed, is simply not healthy, no matter how good it tastes. Five hundred thousand people a year die of heart attacks in this country. High fat levels are the primary factor in the majority of those deaths. Do you love the taste of fat enough to die for it or, worse, to allow your child to die from it?

Of course not. And it doesn't have to be that way. Remember, we're not saying "no" to fat. We're just saying "not as much." That statement sums up our entire approach to diet. It's not a question of no sweets, no treats, and no fats. Moderation is the key, or as they say in the beer ads, it's knowing when to say when. It also involves developing an awareness of what kinds of foods are encouraged, what kinds should be avoided, and what kinds can be substituted for those that are too high in fat.

To trim the fat out of your child's diet, you will need to look not just at individual foods, but at all the foods — the diet as a whole — that your child is eating. It is an approach similar to the way we pediatricians normally treat children. Good pediatricians don't look at just the symptoms, they look at the child. As a medical student on rounds, I recall a professor pointing to one patient and saying, "That's a gall bladder." Separating the problem from the person may have been all right in that setting, but not in real life — and certainly not when dealing with real, live children. Good pediatricians don't look at a patient as an earache. They know the whole child, and they know that child's history. They know what medicine the child's allergic to and which he or she has responded well to. They know whether he or she is the kind of child who resists certain flavors of medicine — and they take all of this into consideration when they plan the child's treatment.

It's the same with the diet. It's not a gram of fat or a hamburger or a plate of vegetables. It's part of a program — a whole program designed for your child's well-being. And in this case, as I obviously don't know your child as well as you do, you'll be the judge. What we're after here is an evolution, not a revolution, in your child's eating habits. As we've said before, we don't have an emergency on our hands. That's why you don't see any claims promising four- or six-week cholesterol "cures" on the cover of this book. This is not a crash diet program; this is a prescription for life. Indeed, we could bring your child's cholesterol down quickly and dramatically with a very rigid diet, but chances are strong that your child would promptly reject the diet as soon as the program was completed. We don't want your kid to be like the little girl who was denied candy as a child and grew up to have the biggest sweet tooth in the dorm. Nor do we want to get into the yo-yo syndrome that so many dieters find themselves caught in.

This slow but steady diet-for-life approach is the philosophy of preventive medicine, a cornerstone of pediatrics. Dr. Ken Cooper, the cardiologist who is probably most famous for inspiring Americans to get off the couch and into exercise programs, summed up the problem of cholesterol this way: "If the epidemic of heart disease in this country is ever going to be controlled, it must start with an aggressive preventive approach with our children."

I agree that the problem must be aggressively dealt with nationally. I would only say, as someone who has dealt with children day in and day out for nearly forty years, that the aggressive approach doesn't always work with a stubborn six-year-old. It takes a little common sense, a little give and take, some easy and gentle day-to-day changes, going, for example, from whole milk to 2 percent milk and then 1 percent milk.

That's the way to do it, in my view, and this is why I feel parents play such an important role in pediatrics. To get back to the earache example, the reason I knew that I shouldn't prescribe a grape-flavored medicine is that Jimmy's mom reminded me that he had spit out the grape-flavored stuff but loved that bubble-gum-flavored medicine we had given him. The same principles work with diet. You know whether your child will more easily accept a fudgecicle or a dish of sherbet as a substitute for ice cream. And if you don't, you'll find out quickly enough!

To make these kinds of choices, you have to understand a little about nutrition and its role in lowering cholesterol levels. Again, the difference in treating high cholesterol levels as opposed to the common aches and ailments of childhood is the response time. With an earache or a sore throat we want to work fast, to give immediate relief. High cholesterol levels and heart disease are a silent but long-term threat, and we advocate a gradual, long-term program, involving these basic guidelines:

1. Eat less high-fat food, especially foods high in saturated fat.
2. Replace part of saturated fat with unsaturated fat in the diet.
3. Eat less high-cholesterol food.
4. Eat foods high in complex carbohydrates (starch and fiber).
5. Reduce weight, if overweight.
6. Be active.

The last two guidelines will be covered in later chapters. The other dietary recommendations are what we will focus on now.

DIET: STEP ONE TO LOWERING YOUR CHILD'S CHOLESTEROL LEVEL

Let's talk about *your* diet for a moment. How will a change in your child's diet affect it? In two words, it shouldn't. Your child shouldn't be expected to eat a different menu from everyone else in the family, nor should you be expected to prepare separate meals for everybody in the house. It's not as if your child has been diagnosed as having diabetes and has to be placed on a special and separate diet from you and the rest of your family. This is an everyday diet for everyone. It's not exotic, not faddist, and not filled with trendy entrees or ingredients. It's a proven prescription, and best of all, it's one you don't have to go to a pharmacy to fill. Everything you need to lower your child's cholesterol level is available at your local supermarket.

I mentioned those six-week "cures" earlier. I don't call this "Dr. Reiman's Reduce-Your-Child's-Cholesterol-Level-Now!" diet for two reasons. First of all, the payoff is long-term, as we've said. Second, this is not a diet I invented during a summer vacation. It's a variation on one of the most sound and sensible diets ever developed: the Step One diet of the American Heart Association (AHA), a proven program that has been used successfully by millions of adults. The difference is that we're going to look at it in more detail, and with an eye toward the realities of child physiology—and psychology.

Following the Step One diet and our other suggestions will result in measurable improvements. Although there are individual differences, the cholesterol level of the average child or adult begins to drop after two to three weeks on the Step One diet. In our own experience, the average we've been able to achieve is a 15 percent drop in total cholesterol; that translates into a 30-point drop for a child with a high cholesterol level of 200. And as it's generally believed that for every 1 percent drop in total cholesterol we may reduce the likelihood of a heart attack by at least 2 percent, you may be reducing your child's chance of a heart attack in later life by 30 percent.

Keep in mind that the amount of decrease depends on how high your child's cholesterol is to begin with, the reduction in saturated fats actually achieved in the diet, and the responsiveness of your child to the diet—because we are all different.

Still, we can safely say that this diet works, and here's why. The basic goal behind the Step One diet is a reduction in total fats, especially saturated fats (we'll explain the difference later) and cholesterol, from their currently unacceptable levels.

How did we arrive at such unacceptable levels in the first place? Partially because of changes in our lifestyle and eating habits over the last century, and partially because of misconceptions about diet as it pertains to fat and cholesterol. Two examples:

Misconception: "If my daughter doesn't drink enough milk,

or if we switch to low-fat milk, she won't get enough calcium to grow properly. Doesn't she need a quart of milk a day?"

No — and no. First, the amount of calcium is essentially the same in whole milk and low-fat milk. Second, the daily recommended requirement of calcium for toddlers — 800 milligrams a day — would be met by three 8-ounce glasses of milk, even if the child ate nothing else the entire day. Assuming your child does eat some green vegetables (a rich source of calcium) on an average day, then she or he needs only two glasses of milk — about half a quart — to meet that 800-milligram target. A supervised low-fat diet does not affect growth. By eliminating that one glass of milk, and by switching to a low-fat milk, not only are you still meeting your child's daily calcium needs, but you've also cut out 26 grams of fat a day.

Misconception: "I know that red meat and eggs have a lot of cholesterol. But cookies and pies are OK — they're just sugar!"

They may not have high cholesterol levels, but cookies and pies are loaded with fat — and the worst kind, at that. People think that if a package of chocolate chip cookies say "cholesterol-free" (as the labels of many baked products do), it's practically a health food. Wrong. The biggest danger in your child's diet isn't cholesterol, but fat — specifically, saturated fat (which, as we'll explain, can help increase the level of LDL in your child's arteries). When we say *fat*, most people think of greasy cheeseburgers, but a dry cookie may contain more saturated fat than an extra-lean hamburger, because it contains more of the wrong kinds of vegetable oils.

With such common misconceptions and lack of awareness, it's no surprise that the average American child's diet — compared with the recommended AHA Step One diet — looks like the one in Table 4.

I'm not sharing this discrepancy with you to depress us

Table 4. Children's Diets[a]

	Current	Recommended[b] (AHA Step One diet)
Total fat (%)	37	30
Polyunsaturated fat (%)	6	10
Monounsaturated fat (%)	14	10–15
Saturated fat (%)	14	Under 10
Cholesterol (milligrams)	193–296 per day	Less than 300

[a]Infants need fat and cholesterol and should not be put on low-fat diets.
[b]Toddlers aged two and three are transitional and so can consume a more flexible diet, gradually approaching the recommended diet.

both. I think it gives goals and targets for your child's diet. The targets are the recommended levels as established in the Step One diet. Our goal should be to bring your child's diet in line with these percentages, and I'll show you how in a moment.

STEP ONE, STEP-BY-STEP

Maybe you have already learned that your child's cholesterol level is high. If so, dietary therapy should begin in the doctor's office — and may have already begun, in fact, because, as we've said, diet is the basis of our program to lower these levels. Your doctor may already have described a basic program that probably looks something like the AHA program and may have given you a pamphlet about it as well (see Table 5).

The Step One diet is where we begin. We go to the Step Two diet later on, if the cholesterol-lowering effect is not satisfactory.

But remember that a pediatrician's time is very limited. I can tell you from my own experience that I'm lucky if I can give

Table 5. *American Heart Association Diets*

	Step One	Step Two
Total fat (%)	30	30
Saturated (%)	10	Less than 7
Polyunsaturated (%)	Less than 10	10
Monounsaturated (%)	10–15	10–15
Cholesterol (mg/day)	300	200
Carbohydrate (%)	50–60	50–60
Protein (%)	15–20	15–20

my patients ten minutes to sketch out an overall diet, much less the hours needed to fine-tune a program for each individual child, and that doesn't include the time I'd love to spend dispelling myths and misconceptions about kids' nutrition, or answering specific questions about the diet.

So how do we get from the typical diet to the recommended Step One diet? As I said before, gradually. And also by understanding the role of the different nutrient groups — and their sources.

The AHA diet, as you can see in Table 5, is based on recommended percentages of carbohydrates, fats, proteins, and cholesterol in the diet. Although our focus will be on fat and cholesterol, I think it will be helpful to do a quick review of the other components of the diet and their functions in nutrition.

CARBOHYDRATES

Although every calorie consumed by the body is energy (indeed, by definition, a calorie is a measurement of heat, which is energy), carbohydrates are the best and most easily used source of energy for the body. They also serve as organic building blocks for the tissues of the entire body. The best carbohydrate, complex carbohydrate, is found in pasta, cereal, bread, and potatoes.

PROTEIN

Mainly useful for tissue building, protein is made up of various combinations of amino acids. It is not directly related to cholesterol, although many high-protein foods, such as red meat and milk, also have high percentages of fat, which is, of course, closely related to cholesterol.

FAT

Do we need any fat? Yes, but whereas it used to be recommended freely as part of a healthy diet, the debate is now over how *little* people can get away with, especially children.

We *do* need fat to manufacture cell membranes and the protective outer layers of the nervous system, and to produce various hormones. What we don't need it for is the production of plaque.

Of course, we've been talking about "fat" as if there's only one type. There are actually *three* types of fat, each of which varies in its effect on cholesterol levels. I'm sure their names are familiar to you, but I find that there is still understandable confusion about which is which—and why. In the lab, the differences have to do with the molecular structures of the different types of fats. In your kitchen, it's enough to know that one of them (saturated) is harmful in excess, another (monounsaturated) is of questionable benefit, and the third (polyunsaturated) is clearly an important part of our diet.

Saturated Fat. Saturated fat is the one that should be avoided in excess. If fat is the culprit in high cholesterol levels, saturated fat is public enemy number one. Where do we find it? In too many of the foods that we eat too much of, I'm afraid: animal foods (meat and poultry), dairy products, and the oils used in baking (coconut, palm, and palm kernel oils). Saturated fat is also a product of hydrogenated fat, such as that found in certain margarines.

Monounsaturated Fats. Monounsaturated fats are not harmful — and may even help to lower total blood cholesterol. They are found in the "good" oils — canola, olive, and peanut oil — as well as in avocados, peanuts, and olives.

Polyunsaturated Fats. Polyunsaturated fats are even more likely than monounsaturated fats to help lower total cholesterol levels and may even raise the level of the other "good" lipoprotein, HDL. These fats are found in other "good" oils — safflower, sunflower, cottonseed, corn, and soybean, which are found in margarine — and in the preferred vegetable oils we will recommend.

There's one element left in our dietary chart, one that may not have appeared on a list like this when you were growing up. Its inclusion reflects an awareness of its importance — and its dangers.

Cholesterol. Cholesterol is not a fat. It's not a starch. It's not vegetable or mineral — but make no mistake about it, it *is* animal. In fact, cholesterol is found *only* in animal foods and their by-products, the dairy foods. It is found more in the skin of poultry than in the poultry itself, and in the heavy concentrations in egg yolk — but not at all in egg white. Plant products are entirely cholesterol-free.

What the AHA breakdown also helps us remember is that cholesterol is not one of the fats. That's another one of those common misconceptions, and that's why it's listed separately from the fats in our AHA Step One diet table. However, the various fats do have an impact on blood cholesterol levels. Saturated fat contributes to the accumulation of cholesterol in the blood, by interfering with LDL's ability to get out of the blood and into the cells. In a sense, the LDL is turned away at the "entrance" to the cell and is therefore left to pile up in the bloodstream, eventually causing fatty streaks and plaques. So, by lowering the amount of saturated fat, we improve the body's ability to deal with the HDL–LDL balancing act that we described in the last chapter. You can think of those saturated fats as being the element that can tip the scales in favor of cholesterol-related problems.

Monounsaturated fats are at least a more benign substitute for the saturated fats. Polyunsaturated fats, on the other hand, may actually counter the efforts of the saturated fats to disrupt the LDL balance. They may help open the "cell door" to LDL, getting it *out* of the bloodstream — our principal goal — and into the cells, where it is metabolized into the production of tissues and the expenditure of energy. That's why reducing fat is the *key* to reducing cholesterol levels: By doing so, we enhance the body's ability to use LDL, as opposed to being abused by it.

To make sure that your child isn't getting too much of the wrong kinds of fats — and plenty of the needed right kinds of nutrients — you'll need to keep track of the amount of fat in the diet. That means knowing which foods are lower or higher in which fats. To help you, we've organized this information in two ways. First, at the back of the book, you'll find a detailed and extensive listing of specific foods and their fat content. I urge you to refer to these lists before you plan your meals and before shopping trips. In the rest of this chapter, we'll categorize fat by its content in the various food groups, as well as by types of foods that have received a great deal of attention of late (some of it justified, and some not).

I recommend that you read the rest of this chapter first to gain a general understanding of the food groups and their benefits and risks in affecting cholesterol levels. Then, we'll show you how to develop a plan: a diet for your child and yourself that's lower in fat.

Some people go crazy trying to memorize the percentages and numbers of the nutrient content of different foods. Often, this effort leads to frustration and rejection of the diet plan. I urge you to read about it, so that you can make better choices in planning your diet, but when it comes to actually deciding on this week's shopping list, don't feel compelled to memorize. Refer to the tables at the end of the book; take them with you to the supermarket. These days, it's not uncommon to see young parents or, for that matter, older couples in the aisles making calculations and careful notes before they reach for the shelves. "Am I allowed to eat that, honey?" is a refrain we hear frequently in our supermarket. I can't help wondering whether, if those people of my age group had been raised on a diet like this as children, they would be asking that question. I think their choices would be second nature, as I'm sure planning this diet will become for you.

FAT AND THE FOOD GROUPS

You don't go to a supermarket and buy carbohydrates. We have to begin to look at our foods as foods, not chemicals or abstract nutrients on a chart. And we'll do this by viewing the food we eat along the lines of the old four food groups that you learned about in your school health class. Keep in mind that, although there is always talk among nutritionists about reclassifying food into new and different groups, the traditional groupings — as well as some important subdivisions — are sufficient for our purposes here and may even be more practical, as most supermarkets are organized roughly along these lines.

I do think it's important to remember this, though. I'm often asked if such-and-such a food is essential or should be totally avoided in a child's diet. No matter what the food, my answer is "no." There is no one food that must be eaten, nor any one food that must *never* be eaten. What's important is not one meal, one dessert, one binge, or even the food eaten during one week or month, but the overall balance over months and years. Each of the food groups, and the different kinds of foods that make up a diet, contributes something, but that doesn't mean that each food within that group is good for your child — specifically, for your child's cholesterol levels. Here are ways to get the most nutrition, with the least fat and cholesterol, out of each food group.

MEATS AND POULTRY

I sometimes wonder, "If the great American dinner hadn't become big, thick steak swimming in gravy and surrounded by tiny portions of vegetables and maybe some buttery mashed potatoes, would cholesterol levels be such a big problem in this country?" My suspicion is that they wouldn't be. Don't misunderstand: There's nothing inherently wrong with steak or roasts or even ground beef; they do contribute protein and other essential vitamins and minerals to your child's diet. It's the portions we serve and the cuts we buy that are the problem.

Forty years ago, if I had made a recommendation to a

mother that she cut back on red meat for her child, I would very likely have been branded a pediatric heretic. The old thinking, which I remember hearing in my medical school nutrition lectures, was that there should be meat on the table most days of the week. You couldn't get too much protein, especially for growing bodies. Grain, vegetables, and legumes were fine, but they were definitely supporting actors.

The new thinking in nutrition, carried to an extreme, is that meat, chicken, and fish are *out* as main courses. Vegetables, fruits, grains, and legumes are in.

We believe that the truth lies somewhere in between. The right place for meat and poultry is neither in nor out, but located a bit off-center on your child's plate. Here are some meaty tips for getting the most benefits from those foods, and the least fat.

RED MEATS

- Stop thinking of meat as the centerpiece of your child's dinner. Start thinking in terms of no more than 3-ounce servings — about the size of a deck of cards — and start increasing the portions of vegetables, starch, and salads. We're not saying to eliminate meat; just serve it more judiciously. A half portion contains half the fat and sufficient protein for your child's needs.
- Choose "lean" or "extra-lean" cuts of meat. These have reduced fat content because meat producers have changed feeding methods, slaughter animals at a younger age, and take greater care in trimming the fat.
- Buy "select" grades rather than "choice" because they have less fat.
- Trim away all visible fat before serving.
- Put limits on luncheon meats and hot dogs — and don't

fry anything. By *limits*, we mean that you can serve it one day if you make up for it the next or even if you substitute another food the same day (you'll see how in a moment).

- Some people think veal is somehow better than beef. Not true. Veal is a little lower in fat, but a little higher in cholesterol. Again, how low in fat it is depends on the cut of the meat. Look for leaner cuts here as well.
- A way to remember which are lower in fat is to choose meats whose names end in *round* or *loin*, because they are leaner.
- Although most meats are OK in smaller servings, I do think these should be avoided as much as possible: corned beef, brisket, club and rib steak, rib roast, breast of lamb, breast of veal, spare ribs, bacon, sausage, organ meats such as liver, deviled ham, beef frankfurters, and cold cuts such as bologna or salami. I know, there are a lot of your favorites on that list—maybe even things you grew up eating. But these processed meats contain 60 to 80 percent fat, mostly saturated, as opposed to lean cuts of beef, which have as little as 30 percent. The organ meats (e.g., liver) are relatively low in fat but very high in cholesterol.

POULTRY

In general, I recommend that you choose poultry—except duck and goose—over beef and pork because, without the skin, they are generally 60 percent lower in saturated fats. However, I think that poultry, like red meat, should be served not as a main course, but as a tasty side dish.

- To get the benefits of poultry, remove the skin when you serve it. It doesn't seem to matter much if you remove it before or after cooking, but remove it you must, because a skinless chicken breast has about *half* the calories and fat of an unskinned breast.

- As with meat, cut away all visible fat.
- As with preparation of all types of food, avoid frying. Fried chicken may be finger-licking good, but it's really artery-clogging bad.
- Choose plain poultry over "self-basting" birds, which have often been injected with oils and high-salt broth.

FISH

Everyone seems to agree that fish is good in the diet, but there are some murky waters here. It is true that most fish is lower in saturated fat than meat and poultry, but certain fish are better than others:

- Choose bluefish, mackerel, salmon, and albacore and bluefin tuna.
- Shellfish are extremely low in fat, especially saturated fat. The amount of cholesterol, however, varies. Lobster is high: a one-and-a-half-pound lobster has about 140 milligrams of cholesterol, nearly half your child's recommended daily allowance. Clams are about average at about 40 milligrams per dozen. A three-and-a-half-ounce serving of Alaska king crab has only 42 milligrams. As far as everyone's favorite shellfish, shrimp, is concerned, the news is mixed: Twelve average-sized shrimp have 130 milligrams of cholesterol but are very low in fat.
- Like oat bran, omega-3 fatty acids got a lot of media attention a few years ago. The truth about them is that they can lower cholesterol and may help reduce atherosclerosis. It is also true that these omega-3 fatty acids are

present in fish. However, the amounts are very small. So my advice on omega-3 is not to eat fish because of this peripheral nutrient. Eat it because of its other, more established nutritional values.

Table 6 provides some examples of just how low the saturated fat content of fish can be, but notice also how widely the cholesterol count may vary.

DAIRY

Because dairy products are such a basic and yet controversial part of your child's diet, they deserve special consideration. Let's start with some basic guidelines:

- Use dairy products with 1 percent or less fat. This doesn't mean that only 1 percent of their total calories are fat. In fact, in 1 percent milk, 22 percent of the *calories* are fat, but as you'll see later when we talk about how to calculate fat content, that's not bad!

Table 6. Fish (per 3½-oz. Cooked Portion)

Fish	Grams of total fat	Grams of saturated fat	Milligrams of cholesterol
Anchovy	9.7 (42%)	2.2 (9.4%)	—
Herring	11.5 (51%)	2.6 (11.5%)	77
Tuna (bluefin)	6.3 (31%)	1.6 (8.0%)	49
Snapper	1.7 (12%)	0.4 (2.8%)	47
Swordfish	5.1 (30%)	1.4 (8.0%)	50
Lobster	0.6 (6%)	0.1 (0.9%)	72
Clam	2.0 (12%)	0.2 (1.2%)	67
Shrimp	1.1 (10%)	0.3 (2.7%)	130

• People think yogurt is health food. It can be, but it can also be fat food. I recommend that you choose nonfat or low-fat yogurt, of which there is now a wide selection.

• Milk and cheese are special cases, and we'll get to them in a minute, but certain kinds of milk and dairy products should be avoided: chocolate milk, cream, sour cream, evaporated whole milk, cream cheese, ice cream, butter, and shortening. Limit egg yolks. I know that these are most of your child's favorite things; it's the stuff that makes other foods creamier and sweeter. The sad truth is that all of these products are high in fat. The good news is that they can be easily replaced by low-fat and nonfat alternatives. Even the cream in your coffee can be replaced by evaporated skim milk.

MILK: THE SPECIAL CASE

Milk—pure, wholesome, white—almost seems to symbolize childhood in all its innocence (Table 7). You may have heard that milk is the perfect food, that it has everything your child needs. I hate to break the news to you, but it's not all it's cracked up to be, and pediatricians have known this for a long time. So why haven't we advised parents to cut out whole milk? Because most would simply refuse to believe we were serious! Their perceptions of milk's essential goodness are so firmly held that they'd look at us as if we've just advised them to have their kids take up smoking.

For children under two, whole milk is fine. As we've said before, we don't recommend any diet modification, with respect to fat, at that age. But over two, it's a different story. Remember that one of the important goals of the Step One diet is to limit fats to 30 percent or less and saturated fats to 10

Table 7. Milk: A Special Case[a]

Type	Calories 8 oz.	Grams of fat	Grams saturated fat[b]	Milligrams of cholesterol
Whole milk	150	8.2 (49%)	4.0 (24%)	34
2% fat (by weight)	120	5.0 (37%)	2.5 (18%)	20
1% fat (by weight)	100	2.5 (22%)	1.2 (11%)	10
Skim milk	90	0.4 (4%)	0.2 (2%)	5

[a]Content varies a little by brand.
[b]Saturated fat content is not usually specified. Assume it to be half of the total fat. Drink the 1 percent fat milk. No wonder 2 percent milk tastes so good.

percent or less. Whole milk doesn't make this task very easy. Even so-called 2 percent milk has 37 percent fat, as calories. An 8-ounce glass of whole milk contains over 8 grams of fat—about 50 percent fat! It's one of the highest fat foods you can serve your child.

The solution to the milk problem, however, is really very easy. Simply use 1 percent milk; it contains 22 percent fat, which fits the bill perfectly, and it's still white, pure, and, if not perfect, at least wholesomely low in fat.

CHEESE

Cheese is another food that has fooled parents. They think that because it's neither fish nor fowl, it must be fine. It's not. Most cheeses are very high in saturated fat and cholesterol. Ounce for ounce, in fact, they have as much cholesterol as meat or poultry—and even more saturated fat. Even part-skim-milk and low-fat cheeses may not be lower in fat than red meat. However, that doesn't mean cheese should not be a part of your child's diet. It's the fat content of the whole meal that counts. Lower-fat cheese combined with, say, pasta and tomato sauce add up to a dish that's tasty, nutritious, and very low in fat.

With so many cheeses on the market, it's sometimes hard to generalize. But here are some suggestions:

- Natural and hard cheeses are the highest in saturated fat. Avoid them. Low-fat and imitation cheeses have less fat. Choose them instead.
- Choose low-fat cottage cheese, skim-milk farmer cheese, and pot cheese. These are all very-low-fat and tasty substitutes.

It is a myth that part-skim cheeses are low in fat. Made from both skim milk and whole milk, they are lower, but not low, as Table 8 illustrates.

BUTTER

Maybe we should title this section "Margarine" because it is smart to choose margarine over butter. However, it's not

Table 8. Fat Content of Sample Cheeses

Cheese	Calories	Grams of fat	Percentage of fat
Mozzarella, whole milk, 1 oz.	80	6	68
Mozzarella, part-skim, 1 oz.	72	4.5	56
Ricotta, whole milk, 4 oz.	216	16	53

easy—at least not when you're in the supermarket, confronted with all those various types of margarine: tub, stick, whipped liquid, light, extra-light, and butter-blend.

How do you make sense of it all? Here are our thoughts on this widespread problem:

- To choose your brand of margarine, just look at two numbers on the label: total fat (you want 6 grams or less of fat per tablespoon) and saturated fat (you want 1 gram or less).

- "Transmonounsaturated fatty acids." It may be clumsy to say, but it's not difficult to evaluate these new additives. They're produced as a result of the hydrogenation process, which is done to help make some margarine firmer. The harder the margarine, the more of these transmonounsaturated fatty acids they contain.

  Although they sound nasty—and they do act like the saturated fats that raise cholesterol—there's really no need to worry about them. Their effect is negligible. They make for an interesting news story, but they are present in such small quantities that they don't make much difference in your child's diet.

- One last tip about margarine: You might simply try using less. Have you ever seen the way some people butter up their rolls or bagels? It's more butter than bread and probably packs as much cholesterol wallop as if you simply slapped a piece of steak on your breakfast roll instead.

  Try putting less on your child's food—definitely less butter, and maybe even less margarine as well. Your child—and you—might find that bread can still taste pretty good without it, or with less. And as always, this kind of change can be made gradually—a breakfast a week, perhaps. You may even switch to jam or apple butter (no fat).

CEREALS, BREADS, PASTAS, STARCHES

Dieters used to think that a slice of bread was applied directly to your hips. Even today, when I discuss diet with the parents of overweight children, one of their first impulses is to cut down on bread. They're so wrong. Grains are great. In fact, bread *is* diet food. A single slice has only about 100 calories (it's the butter that provides the fat and the calories).

As far as cholesterol in the diet is concerned, grains supply fiber, which reduces cholesterol (see below), and fiber is found mainly in oat bran, barley, and dried beans. Our suggestions on this important food family are the following:

- In general, you should include plenty of these carbo-hydrate-rich foods in your child's diet: rice, pasta, kidney beans, and lentils, in addition to the ever-present bread and potatoes. Besides supplying heart-healthy fiber, they are excellent sources of vitamins and minerals, and they're filling, too.
- We think of cereals as junk food. They are if they're heavily sweetened or mixed with fatty nuts and granola. Contrary to what "hippies" and health food faddists in the 1960s and 1970s thought, granola is not health food. Its bottom line is that, although it contains only 70 milligrams of cholesterol and is low in saturated fat, it contains a hefty 45 percent of total fat. But "good" breakfast cereals are very low in fat. Choose

oatmeal and bran cereals over the frosted brand of the
month.
- Choose rye, whole wheat, and pumpernickel bread over
white. They have less fat because lower-fat oils are
used to bake them.

A Few Words about Fiber and Bran

Is bran heart-healthy or heart-hype? A University of Texas
Southwestern Medical Center study showed that oat bran,
given as part of the Step One diet, helped reduce average
cholesterol by 7 percent and increased HDL. Other studies
have found similar benefits from bran. And yet, a study that
received widespread attention in 1990 seemed to demythify oat
bran, showing that the reductions in cholesterol among people
who ate oat bran was partially explained by the fact that they
had lowered the fat content in other parts of their diet. In other
words, oat bran's contribution may have been misleading. As
usual, the truth probably lies somewhere in between. I would
caution you against thinking that feeding yourself or your child a
dozen oat bran muffins a day makes you immune to high
cholesterol. I do, however, agree that bran and fiber are essential
parts of your child's diet. Let's look at the relationship.

Fiber is the indigestible cell wall of plants. It's found
mainly in grains, but also in fruits and vegetables, as well as in
dried beans, peas, and other legumes. Bran is the indigestible
but fiber-rich outer layer or kernel of the "cereal" grains, such
as oat, wheat, rice, and barley. As it is not digestible, fiber
remains in the intestine, where it absorbs the bile acids manufactured by the liver from cholesterol. This is the body's way of
disposing of excess cholesterol in the stool. So, fiber, by holding

onto those bile acids that would normally be returned to the
liver to make new cholesterol, acts as a sort of cholesterol
"blocker."

The bottom line is that getting your child to eat more fiber,
especially bran and especially in cereals, will help bring cholesterol down. Americans have diets that are too low in fiber. I
recommend that you try to include 10 to 15 grams of fiber a day
in your child's diet. (Table 9 shows you which foods can help you
meet that goal.)

Table 9. Fiber

	Ounces of sample foods necessary to supply 10 grams of fiber
Cereals	
Bran itself	1.1
Rolled oats	3.9
Grape-Nuts	3.2
Shredded Wheat	2.9
Breads	
Whole wheat	0.9 per slice
Rye	1.1
White	0.9
Vegetables	
Green beans	14.7
Broccoli	16.5
Carrots	16.8
Lettuce	22.0
Fruits	
Apples	10.2
Strawberries	17.0
Bananas	19.6
Peaches	2.1
Cantaloupe	30.2

However, I also recommend that you not be distracted by bran. It's a helpful but not essential adjunct to the diet. Your primary goal should still be to reduce the amount of dietary fat in your child's meals, especially saturated fat.

BAKED GOODS

Some people would have you believe that croissants, biscuits, and butter rolls are synonymous with the whole-grain breads and cereals we just discussed. Sorry. Most contain a lot of saturated fat, in the form of egg yolks, cream, and butter. Avoid these "fat breads" and choose hard rolls, pita bread, bagels, French or Italian bread, breadsticks, matzos, and crisps instead. (But again, go easy on the butter or you'll defeat the whole purpose!)

FRUITS AND VEGETABLES

This section is very brief. Why? Because, you'll recall, plant products have no cholesterol and very little fat. So, these foods should be emphasized heavily in your child's diet, with a few cautions:

- Avoid butter or sour cream toppings.
- Serve your vegetables raw or steamed.
- Avoid fruits canned in heavy syrup.
- Use fruits without added sugar.
- A recommendation: Consider using fruit as a substitute for sweets (see our substitution tables for more specific recommendations).

SALADS

You can do a lot with salad—a lot of good, and a lot of harm, from a nutritional point of view. Chef salads that are bathed in heavy dressings, garnished with strips of ham and sprinkled with bacon bits are not exactly what I'd call heart healthy. Indeed, most commercial dressings are 90% fat—and many also contain added egg, cream, or cheese. Consider that two tablespoons of Ranch, blue cheese, or Russian dressing can add 150 calories and about as much fat as a *pint* of whole milk.

So here are some suggestions on how to make the versatile salad an ally in the fight against fat in your child's diet:

- Place dressing on the side and use as little as possible. Choose low-fat, low-oil dressings, but be sure to read the label.
- Try making your own vinegar-and-oil dressing, but make sure the oils are the ones lowest in saturated fat: canola, safflower, or sunflower. Flavor with herbs or flavored vinegar.
- "Stretch" a commercial dressing by adding a low-fat ingredient such as lemon juice, nonfat yogurt, or pureed tomato.
- Leave out the oil completely. Instead, experiment with flavors such as lemon or lime juice, pureed tomato, nonfat yogurt, apple juice, mustard, garlic, herbs, or peppers.
- This has nothing to do with fat and cholesterol, but it is nutritionally smart to choose romaine, Boston lettuce, spinach, or other forms of lettuce over the most common, iceberg, which is low in any nutrients whatsoever.

SOUPS AND BROTH

There's nothing like a piping-hot bowl of soup on a cold day. Like milk, it's one of those foods that seems synonymous with wholesomeness and good nutrition. By giving your child a bowl of soup, you must be doing something right, right? Not necessarily. My advice:

- Avoid creamy, "chunky," or so-called hearty soups.
- Choose clear broth soups with rice, noodles, and vegetables. Better yet, if you have time, prepare your own soups, being careful to remove all fat.
- Bring on the broth. Broth or "stock," the liquid that results from boiling meats, fish bones, or vegetables, has long been used as the basis for soups, stews, and sauces.

I recommend broth as a low-fat ingredient for all of the above. Try to avoid store-bought broths — the kind that come in cubes, cans, or powders — as they are high in salt and other flavor additives. If you use canned stock, you can remove the fat by chilling the can and then spooning off the solid fat on top.

SNACKS

Perhaps you're surprised we even include "Snacks" as a heading. You shouldn't be. Remember that we're working toward a realistic, not a rigid, diet, a diet of modification, not total elimination.

Junk food, as I tell parents, is all right occasionally, but a junk-food diet is not. Your child can splurge from time to time, but simply be aware and compensate. Save the high-fat foods for special occasions like birthday parties; that's when most kids eat ice cream. Trying to stop them is self-defeating. You can't be a police officer with your kids. You've got to give them breathing room: They are kids, and they want to do what other kids do. So, from time to time, let them.

Remember that no one meal makes or breaks a diet. We'll talk more about how to achieve this balance in our chapter on compliance. For now, here's our advice on how to minimize the damage from those inevitable snack attacks:

- Avoid cookies, pies, ice cream, potato and corn chips, and nuts. Instead, try serving more fruits and vegetables, raisins, low-fat frozen yogurt, unbuttered popcorn, gingersnaps, homemade oatmeal cookies, and — believe it or not — angel food cake, a heavenly addition to the list of sweet snacks that your child can eat. They're all lower in fat and, don't forget, high in taste. Try 'em. You might be surprised how much your kids will like 'em.

- I'm often asked about the new no-fat, no-cholesterol cookies and cakes and the frozen desserts made with the fat substitute Simplesse. Are they a safe substitute all the time? As far as fat and cholesterol are concerned, they are, provided that they are low in both. However, they are high in sugar, and even in salt. They're an adjunct — a treat — not a main part of the diet. They're an improvement over the real high-fat McCoy, but you wouldn't want your child living on them.

4

How to Build
a Diet That Works

We've looked at how individual foods stack up in terms of their fat and cholesterol content. Now, we have to put it all together. We have to organize all of this information in order to develop a diet that you and your child can live with.

My purpose in this chapter is to give you the tools to help you build a program for eating that, if properly followed, *will* lower your child's cholesterol — without making your child feel different or singled out. I offer as proof the families that I serve in my pediatric practice. Since we first started cholesterol testing in 1985, I've worked with literally thousands of families developing programs to lower their children's cholesterol. The results speak for themselves. Without the use of drugs or even diet supplements, we have managed to achieve an average reduction in total cholesterol level of 15 percent. That translates, for example, into a reduction from a high 200 to a safe 170. Not only is our batting average a good one — having a success rate that's consistent with the results of other programs and practitioners who use approaches similar to ours — but it also dramatically reduces the chance that our children will have heart attacks in future years: an estimated 30 percent reduction in risk.

We're equally proud of the fact that our parents have achieved these results without pills or surgery. The results were primarily accomplished by implementing lifestyle changes, particularly in diet. Of course, *diet* is a dirty word, and admittedly, it's not a very fair business. Some kids can live on a diet of hot fudge sundaes and still stay skinny, whereas others cannot. Similarly, some people—children as well as adults—can eat huge amounts of high-fat and high-cholesterol foods and not have high cholesterol readings. Why is that? Very simply, it's because these people are better able to clean cholesterol—in the form of LDL—out of their bloodstreams.

Of course, such people are rare. For most, your child included, eating a diet lower in fat is the single most important step toward lowering cholesterol levels. We all have to work with our own genetic makeup. Many parents assume that because a high cholesterol level may be hereditary, it must be as impossible to change as the color of their child's eyes. Except in the rarest of cases, this is absolutely not true. Almost any child will benefit from dietary modification.

Again, I think of parents of my patients who've achieved terrific results without drastic or dramatic changes in their lifestyle. Furthermore, they did not have to become amateur dieticians and spend all of their time counting carbohydrates and preparing special foods.

It's important to emphasize the simplicity of our plan. Most of the diet books on the best-seller list espouse very sound principles and programs, many of them similar to the ones you'll read here. But often, these diets don't work. Why not? Because people get frustrated. Dieting seems to take too much effort and concentration, too much calculation, and too much willpower.

I'd like to think that our approach is different, maybe because it's based on insights gained not only from the laboratory, but from life — from knowing parents, from being a parent, and from working with both parents and their kids. We know that you and your child are not going to spend your lives counting fat grams. That's why we use these diets and calculations only as a stepping stone to our ultimate goal, which is a diet that you can understand, are comfortable with, and don't have to become overly preoccupied with planning.

The arithmetic involved in this diet is so easy that your children could probably do it themselves, and the principles underlying it are sound. As we've said, this is not a radical diet; it's a moderate, commonsense program for eating. It's been accepted and approved by some of the most reliable authorities on nutrition in the country, and it's been used successfully by millions of adults to lower their cholesterol levels.

The difference here, of course, is that we're not dealing with adults. We're dealing with your child, and children have different nutritional needs from yours and mine. Quantifying that difference, in terms of calories, is where we start building our diet.

The benchmark is daily caloric expenditure. Calories, as you probably know, are the measurement of the energy provided by food in the diet. Kids need enough caloric energy food to grow, to develop, and just to be kids! Someone who calls a child "a bundle of energy" is not far off the mark. So we have to make sure that children's caloric requirements are met. Those requirements differ from child to child, but for our purposes, we can come up with a general estimate of your child's caloric expenditure, first just by his or her age (see Table 10).

What do we mean in the Table 10 footnote by "degree of activity"? It's hard to measure precisely. It's quite subjective, in fact, but look at it this way: If your child is spending nine hours

72 CHAPTER 4

Table 10. Total Calories Needed by Your Child

Age (years)		Calorie range	Average[a]
1–3		900–1,800	1,300
4–6		1,300–2,300	1,700
7–10		1,650–3,300	2,400
11–14	(males)	2,000–3,700	2,700
	(females)	1,500–3,000	2,200
15–18	(males)	2,100–3,900	2,800
	(females)	1,200–3,000	2,100
19–22	(males)	2,500–3,300	2,900
	(females)	1,700–2,500	2,100

[a]Naturally, these are just averages that vary with body build, degree of activity, and whether you wish your child to reduce or add weight.
Source: Recommended Dietary Allowances, National Academy of Sciences, 10th ed., 1989.

a day playing Nintendo, that's "light activity." If she or he is running around outside with friends, playing ball or riding a bike, that's "very active." If she or he plays all afternoon and watches a little TV in the evening, that's "moderate activity." So, as an example, inactive seven-year-olds need only about 1,650 calories a day, but seven-year-olds who play soccer with their friends all day will burn closer to 3,300—and are doing themselves a world of good in other ways as well.

Compare Table 10 with Table 11. A four-year-old who weighs 40 pounds and is moderately active would require a daily average of 1,700 calories, according to Table 10. According to Table 11, a moderately active 40-pound four-year-old requires 41 calories per pound, that is, 41 times 40, or 1,640 calories. The results from Tables 10 and 11 are quite similar.

Sometimes, the differences in activity levels are seasonal.

Table 11. *Total Daily Calories*

Another way of figuring your child's needs for calories is based on *your estimate* of his or her degree of activity. You may increase or reduce the recommendations by 10 percent in order to promote weight gain or reduction.

	Calories per pound of body weight		
Age (years)	Lightly active	Moderately active	Very active
1–3	36	45	54
4–6	33	41	49
7–10	26	32	39
11–14 (males)	20	25	30
(females)	17	22	26
15–18 (males)	17	21	25
(females)	15	18	22

Source: Calculated from data in Recommended Dietary Allowances, National Academy of Sciences, 10th ed., 1989, p. 3.

Even the most rambunctious of children spend more sedentary time during the school year, behind a desk, than they do in the summer. Although it's a good idea to be aware of these differences (and you may want to compensate for them as you become more familiar with this diet plan), I think you can start by estimating the daily average total caloric expenditure of your child, based on age. The figure will not be absolutely precise, but it will be precise enough for our purposes here.

Now that you have a total number of calories, let's look at how to allocate those calories. Our program is based on the American Heart Association (AHA) Step One diet, which recommends that no more than 30 percent of daily calories should be in the form of fat, and that no more than a third of those should be saturated fat. (The rest of the percentages, as you'll remember from Table 5 in Chapter 3, are 50 to 60 percent carbohydrate and 15 to 20 percent protein.)

Fat is measured in grams. To make sure your child's diet doesn't exceed the AHA maximum of 30 percent fat calories per day, you may start by counting fat *grams*. That's easy; they're usually listed on the labels of most foods. But how do you know how much is too much?

There's an easy formula for calculating the target number of fat grams for your child's diet. It's based on the fact that every gram of fat is equal to nine calories, and our goal, as stated earlier, is that fat *calories* should not exceed 30 percent of *total* calories. But you don't have to worry about a lot of multiplication or calculation of percentages with this formula. Simply take the total daily caloric recommendations for your child (listed on Tables 10 and 11), drop the final zero, and divide by 3. Let's assume your child needs 1,500 calories per day. Dropping the zero leaves 150. Dividing that by 3 gives us 50 grams of fat per day. That's your daily target.

I like to think of the daily target as an allotment. In other words, you have 50 grams of fat (or 450 fat calories) in the dietary bank account that your child can eat — or spend — each day. We begin to construct our diet just as you would figure out a budget. At first, you may find some surprises in the fat "cost" of various food items, such as a glass of whole milk, which — parents are often horrified to hear — contains over 8 grams of fat. A child who drinks three glasses of whole milk has used up half of his or her fat allotment for the entire day — not what I'd call a bargain. But there are pleasant surprises as well.

Eventually, you'll learn to use these fat grams as easily as you handle dollars and cents. And just as you've probably learned that being careful with your money is the way to make sure that you'll have what you need when you need it, the same is true of your child's dietary budget. You'll want to be prudent in your purchases and not "blow" all of the grams of fat on something frivolous.

However, you can still allow your child to have some fun and enjoy some of the fatty foods that kids inevitably crave, and that your child will want to eat, if only to be like other kids. As responsible adults, we occasionally splurge on a vacation, a new dress, or a new set of golf clubs, provided we've planned for it and have set aside the money. Use the same principles with your dietary budget. If your child eats a bit too much ice cream at the birthday party on Saturday, you can balance it out on Sunday. If she or he had 60 grams of fat the day you visited Grandma's house instead of the allotted 50 grams, don't panic; don't think that the diet is blown or that your child's cholesterol level is rising before your eyes. And most of all, don't give up the program! Simply make sure that your child eats a total of only 40 grams of fat on Monday. It's easy, if you take the time to plan, and if you understand the fat value of various foods.

And by the way, although some say a dollar doesn't go very far these days, you'll be amazed at how much good taste and nutrition you can get with only a few grams of fat. Take the previous example. If you have to restrict your child to 40 grams of fat because he "overdrew" the day before, you need not sentence her or him to twenty-four hours of bread and water. Far from it. At the end of this book, you'll find a comprehensive listing of the fat content, expressed in grams, of many of the most common foods. To give you a sense of what kind of low-fat bargains you can cook up, consider this lunch: a turkey-breast-and-lettuce sandwich, carrot sticks, a glass of milk with 1 percent milkfat, and a slice of angel food cake with chocolate frosting. How many grams of fat do you think this meal contains? Thirty? Twenty? Ten? Keep going. That delicious and nutritious lunch contains a total of 7.8 grams of fat. Here's the breakdown:

Food	Grams of fat
3 ounces of turkey breast	0.9
2 slices of bread	1.8
Lettuce	0
$\frac{1}{3}$ cup of carrot sticks	0
1 cup of 1% milk	2.6
Angel food cake	0.1
Chocolate frosting	2.4
Total	7.8

Now you can begin to read labels and intelligently plan a diet that will lower your child's cholesterol level and keep it low. We'll talk specifically about how to read labels in the next chapter, but before you go racing to the supermarket, let's take a closer look at the whole concept of what makes a healthy diet.

For purposes of simplicity, we've been talking about fat grams, but as you'll recall from our earlier discussions, it's not just the total number of fat grams that matters. It's especially the grams of saturated fat. Also, we need to be aware of cholesterol in animal foods, which are usually expressed in milligrams (mg), and to keep in mind that we are not just counting up fat grams without any thought about the balance and quality of the foods they represent.

A word about those four food groups. To refresh your memory, here they are:

1. Meat, poultry, fish, eggs, beans, and nuts
2. The milk group
3. The fruit and vegetable group
4. The grain group

The idea of organizing all foods into "families" as a way of planning a diet became most popular after World War II, when the U.S. Department of Agriculture (USDA) instituted a widespread educational campaign throughout the media and in our schools, promoting this notion of the four food groups. It was a fine concept. The problem was that, based on the prevailing nutritional wisdom of the day, the USDA favored some of the families over others. Americans — particularly growing children — were urged to eat plenty of servings of red meat, whole dairy products, and eggs.

I mentioned earlier in this book that heart disease — and the high cholesterol levels associated with it — are, in a way, a penalty of affluence. This idea was borne out by independent research conducted soon after the USDA campaign was launched. Researchers found that poorer Americans living in rural areas, whose diet consisted primarily of vegetables and starch (the old name for complex carbohydrates), had a lower incidence of heart attacks than middle- and upper-class Americans, who were following the red meat, egg, and dairy dictums of the USDA.

Those who followed the recommendations paid for it — and we're all still paying for it. Indeed, I firmly believe that the high level of heart disease in this country — and the enormous social costs that are associated with it — is attributable in part to the well-intentioned but misinformed propaganda of our own government. It gave an entire generation a firm, but wrong, idea of what constituted proper nutrition.

The point is that you don't have to spend more money to eat better. And that point leads us to choice of foods, the essence of our diet program. This is where you take the information you've calculated about fat grams and convert it into the actual foods you will put on your child's plate. The choice of those foods is the essence of the diet plan. It's called *substitution*. This is how you get the most for your money — or, in this case, the most food (and nutritional value) for your fat allotment. Substitution simply means that you can select certain foods in the place of others in order to get the most taste and the most nutrition with the least possible fat.

Again, think of it as smart shopping. If you can get two portions of something that "costs" you only 4 grams of fat — instead of one portion that has the same fat cost — you're ahead of the game, just as if you'd taken advantage of a two-for-one deal at a retail store. And in the case of food substitution, it's an even better deal, because the food we substitute is not only "cheaper," it's also of higher quality.

A case in point: Two tablespoons of creamy salad dressing "costs" your child about 16 grams of fat. For half that amount of fat, you might try another nutritious lunch that no child could complain about, if only because it includes yet another dessert:

Food	Grams of fat
Chicken-noodle soup	2.5
English muffin	1.2
Tuna in water	1.7
Dressing, low-fat	0.8
Orange sherbet	1.9
Total	8.1

By substituting a low-fat dressing on the salad at one meal, you have earned an entire lunch for your child, and you still have half the fat grams left over, to spend as you wish.

In the following pages, you'll find lists of recommendations for low-fat, high-nutrition substitutes to help you maintain your balance. You'll find some surprises, and you'll also find some time-honored "truths" about nutrition exposed as the myths that they are. For example, veal is not any better — in terms of fat — than beef, and the difference between the dark and the white meat of chicken is insignificant: about 1 gram in an entire

3-ounce serving of each. And how about this blue-plate special? Choose a broiled, fat-trimmed lean round steak over a broiled club steak, and you'll be saving 39 grams of fat.

These and other insights are some of the benefits of building a diet around substitution, but I think it's important to incorporate some other principles, as well. Although this isn't a handbook for general nutrition and we don't want to get into an argument about the debatable minutiae of trace minerals, we also don't want to focus so much on fat and cholesterol that we lose sight of the larger picture. We do care equally about protein, about carbohydrates, about limiting salt and sugar, and about maintaining a healthy balance of foods. Here are some general thoughts on planning a well-balanced diet for your child:

- There is no agreement among scientists about how much salt is safe, but there is general agreement that the less your child eats, the better. Like fat and calories, much salt (sodium) is hidden in prepared foods. An oft-cited example is that a baked potato has almost no sodium, whereas the same weight in potato chips has nearly 1,000 milligrams. Generally, more than 140 milligrams of sodium per serving is considered high-salt.
- I don't recommend that you altogether ban table sugar from your child's diet. I've known too many kids who were denied sweets and became sugar-crazed adults. Let your child indulge in sweets once in a while, but limit them. Sugar adds unnecessary calories to food and contributes heavily to tooth decay.
- The American Heart Association Step One diet maintains that 15 to 20 percent of your diet should come from protein, and that 50 to 60 percent should come from carbohydrates. This is a perfectly suitable formula for children as well.

- A new spinoff of the old categories of food groups has been developed with new recommendations for the number of servings from each different group. This "food pyramid" (see Figure 1) indicates that we should eat less of the foods at the top point of the pyramid (fats, oils, and sweets) and more of those at the broad bottom (bread, cereal, rice, and pasta).

As reported in the *New York Times*, some food producers (the dairy and meat groups) initially protested because the ranking of foods seemed to give their products a poor dietary image. Eleven months and $855,000 later, a slightly revised pyramid shown in Figure 1 was released by the USDA. Most nutritionists, the U.S. government, and I heartily recommend that you follow this guide in planning your child's diet.

Paying attention to the many recommendations for healthy eating might, if you are not careful, lead you to slip into a repetitious and boring selection of foods. Don't let this happen. Yes, your child could live on a daily diet of turkey or tuna fish, lettuce, and tomatoes, and his or her cholesterol level would probably get lower. But at what cost? Following such a limited diet would sacrifice other important nutrients. So do vary the diet, and try not to let your child get into a pattern of eating the same foods again and again. Introduce a variety of foods and encourage experimentation.

Let's get ready to put your diet into action. Rather than heading into the supermarket and winging it, I recommend that you take a few minutes after reading this chapter to study the substitutions in Table 12. Look for the foods that you normally eat and serve your child. Then see what you can do about eliminating or making substitutions for some of the offenders.

One tip I can give you is this: Rome wasn't built in a day, and neither is a child's low-fat diet. How far you go with these

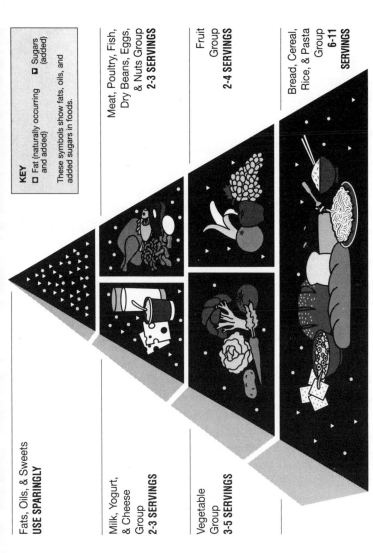

KEY
□ Fat (naturally occurring and added) □ Sugars (added)

These symbols show fats, oils, and added sugars in foods.

Fats, Oils, & Sweets
USE SPARINGLY

Milk, Yogurt, & Cheese Group
2-3 SERVINGS

Meat, Poultry, Fish, Dry Beans, Eggs, & Nuts Group
2-3 SERVINGS

Vegetable Group
3-5 SERVINGS

Fruit Group
2-4 SERVINGS

Bread, Cereal, Rice, & Pasta Group
6-11 SERVINGS

Figure 1. Good Guide Pyramid: A Guide to Daily Food Choices (Courtesy of the U.S. Department of Agriculture, Human Nutrition Information Service)

Table 12. Table of Food Substitutions

Instead of	Use
Breads, cereals, rice, and pasta	
White bread	Whole-grain bread
Chips and crackers	Pretzels, bagel chips, popcorn, and dried fruits
High-fat crackers	Saltines, Rye Krisp, and matzos
Butter rolls and croissants	Low-fat rolls, bagels, and pita bread
Granola-type cereals	Cereals without added granola or nuts
Butter on toast	Jam or jelly
Meats, poultry, fish, eggs, beans, and nuts	
Whole egg	Egg substitute or two egg whites
Regular meat	Lean or extra-lean, well-trimmed, lightly marbled meat
Ground beef	Ground turkey
Poultry with skin	Skinless poultry
Meat in general	"Select" instead of "choice" cuts; smaller portions or a substitution of beans, peas, legumes, or tofu
Hamburger	Work toward leaner beef; "regular" to ground chuck to ground round to ground sirloin
Organ meats	Lean meat, poultry, and fish
Meat sauce	Meatless sauce
Deep-fried chicken	Stir-fried chicken, breadless
Hot dogs, bologna, salami, bacon, and sausage	Tuna in water, turkey or chicken breast, and lean cuts of meat
Canned fish in oil	Canned fish in water
Fried or breaded fish	Broiled, baked, poached, or steam fish without breading or butter
Nuts	Pretzels, popcorn, and bagel chips

(Continued)

Table 12. (Continued)

Instead of	Use
Milk group	
Whole milk	1% or skim milk
Cream or whipped cream	Evaporated skim milk
Sour cream	Low-fat yogurt
Yogurt	Low-fat yogurt
Butter	Tub margarine (stick margarine is more hydrogenated, which raises blood cholesterol levels)
Whole-milk cheeses (American, Swiss, cheddar, or Romano)	Skim-milk or low-fat cheese (2–6 grams of fat per ounce)
Cream cheese	Low-fat cottage cheese
Stick margarine	Tub margarine
Cream soups	Add skim milk to clear soups
Butter on pancakes	Fruit on pancakes
Sour cream dip	Low-fat yogurt dip or salsa
Ice cream	Sherbet or the low-fat desserts
Milkshake	Water or fruit juice
Fruits, oils, and desserts	
Mayonnaise	Low-fat mayonnaise, mustard, and ketchup
Regular salad dressing	No-fat and low-fat dressings
Regular sauces and gravies	Low-fat sauces and marinades
Hydrogenated vegetable oil	Partially hydrogenated vegetable oil
Gravy and fatty sauces	Bouillon and juices
High-fat snacks	Fresh and dried fruits
Buttered popcorn	Unbuttered, "air-popped" popcorn

(Continued)

Table 12. (*Continued*)

Instead of	Use
Store-bought cakes, cookies, doughnuts, or pastry	No-fat cake, angel food cake, graham crackers, fig newtons, and ginger snaps
High-fat desserts such as ice cream or frozen regular yogurt	Fresh fruit, sherbet, low-fat frozen yogurt, and ice milk

Fruits and vegetables

Eat all you want. They contain no cholesterol and virtually no fat. But watch out for added butter, creams, sauces, or cheese. Use fruits without added sugar. Vegetables should be steamed, microwaved, or pan-fried without oil. Be careful with canned vegetables, which may be very high in salt.

substitutions will depend on your own personality, on your child's compliance, and most important, on how high your child's blood cholesterol level is. The diet of a child with a cholesterol level of 160 may require only some fine-tuning, whereas if the cholesterol level is 260, much more aggressive substitution is obviously required.

No matter how fast you hope to reach your goal, start gradually, perhaps by substituting for just one meal per week, or even one food. Many of my patients have introduced themselves and their kids to the substitution method by focusing first on one important yet easily made exchange: Instead of buying whole milk, they buy milk with 2 percent milkfat. By doing that, you can go from 50 percent fat to 35 percent fat, put a little deposit in your dietary bank, and take your first giant step toward using fat-gram counting and substitution to plan a diet that will lower your child's cholesterol now — and for the rest of her or his life.

LOW-FAT COOKING

We've talked about how to trim the fat from your child's diet, but how do we keep it out of your pots and pans? Humans have been using animal fats to flavor their foods since the days when the kitchen was in a cave. It's a tough habit to break, but fortunately, we do have a few fat-busting tricks.

The key to low-fat cooking is the same as the key to low-fat nutrition: substitution. And the key to pleasing your children is making those substitutions gradually. Experiment with some of these suggestions, but go slowly:

- First, get rid of your deep-fat fryer, an all-too-common utensil in the home of families with kids. Deep-fat frying drowns your child's food in liquid fat. Need we say more?
- In pan cooking, use only a small amount of olive oil or, better yet, an oil spray. A dash of the former or a small squirt of the latter can be used to prevent sticking or can be added near the end of the cooking if the recipe calls for some oil. Keep in mind that the sprays contain less than 10 calories and a negligible amount of fat.

    Other common substitutes for oil include chicken stock, a mixture of flavored vinegar with broth or wine, and fresh lemon juice.
- When following recipes, substitute two egg whites for each egg yolk, use only low-fat milk, and, of course, use only the low-fat cuts of meat, poultry, or fish.

5

What's Inside Your Refrigerator?

By now, you should have a good idea of which foods are healthy for your child, and which should be off-limits — or at least to be saved as special treats. The next step is to put smart nutrition into practice. You can begin by examining your pantry, refrigerator, and kitchen cupboards for foods that are high in fat and/ or cholesterol. Some of them have no redeeming nutritional value whatever, so you'll want to banish them; some you may save for treats; still others you may be able to use more often by preparing them differently.

Believe it or not, you won't wind up tossing out everything that tastes good, nor will you feel deprived if you eat a favorite food twice a month instead of twice a week. I can vouch for that: My wife and I performed a kitchen audit in our own home several years ago, and neither of us misses a single ousted item. More important, hundreds of my patients' parents have done the same, and their families are all the healthier for it. So let's get started.

Begin by raiding your refrigerator. It's very likely that you'll have neat rows of eggs in your refrigerator door. The yolks in those innocuous-looking little brown or white ovals account for a full 45 percent of the average American child's cholesterol intake. Therefore, the current recommendation by most nutritionists is that egg yolks be limited to no more than two or three a week. There is no such ban on the protein-rich, cholesterol-free whites, however, and these can be used in place of the yolks called for in many recipes. A good rule of thumb is to replace every yolk with two whites, so if a recipe calls for four eggs, you would use eight whites. But what should be done with all of the leftover yolks? Having grown up during the Depression, I hate to see wasted food, so here are some suggestions: Cooked egg yolks can be fed to the pet dog, who isn't in danger of clogged arteries and whose coat will benefit from the treat, or they can be crumbled into the bird feeder. (Don't try mixing raw yolks into your favorite canine's food: Man's best friend is vulnerable to *Salmonella* bacteria.) Or you can hunt down recipes for homemade hand lotions and hair conditioners that call for egg yolks.

An alternative replacement is egg substitutes, which usually come in convenient, freezable packages resembling milk cartons. These have no cholesterol and can stand in for eggs in virtually any recipe.

Next door to the eggs, no doubt, you'll find the butter. This most popular companion to bread is made up almost entirely of saturated fat and contains 32 milligrams of cholesterol per tablespoon. Although some recipes may cry out for the taste of the real stuff, there are spreads for bread that are lower in fat and cholesterol, namely, the vast array of margarines on the market. Most of these pack a bit more water than fat and are made from vegetable oils, such as sunflower oil, corn oil, safflower oil, and cottonseed oil. Thus they are cholesterol-free.

Let's move on to the dairy area of your fridge to the compartment or shelf where you keep yogurt, cheeses, and such. Despite its health food reputation, yogurt made from whole milk is not a fat bargain: one 8-ounce serving of plain yogurt has over 7 grams of fat. More to the point, 48 percent of its roughly 140 calories is derived from fat, nearly 75 percent of which is saturated. I know that's a lot of numbers to toss around, but here's another: Plain, whole-milk yogurt packs 30 milligrams of cholesterol.

Fortunately, not all yogurts are created equal. The low-fat varieties made from skim milk add up to a much healthier food. In 8 ounces of plain low-fat yogurt, you'll find only 127 calories, less than half a gram of fat and only 5 milligrams of cholesterol. The only catch, and you can barely call it that because the numbers are so good, is that most of the fat is saturated; if that bothers you, there are numerous *nonfat* yogurts to choose from.

Which brings us to cheese, a favorite of youngsters who would probably exist on pizza, nachos, and grilled-cheese sandwiches given the opportunity. Because the different kinds vary widely in amounts of fat, saturated fat, and cholesterol, it is difficult to generalize about cheeses, but let's look at two of the most popular ones among the sneaker set: the mozzarella that adorns pizza and the processed American cheese that usually winds up wedged between two pieces of bread in the broiler. Mozzarella cheese made from whole milk has 90 calories, 7 grams of fat (which boils down to 70 percent calories from fat), and 25 milligrams of cholesterol per 3-ounce serving. Now for American cheese: A single orange square packs as many as 115 calories, 26 milligrams of cholesterol, and 9 grams of fat, more than half of which is saturated.

Get the message? At the same time, you needn't ban cheese completely. In reasonable amounts (an 8-ounce serving once or twice a week), most cheeses are good sources of protein and calcium — both necessary nutrients for growing children.

You may also want to try some of the low-fat and nonfat cheeses that are available.

A close cousin of cheese is cottage cheese, also known as pot cheese. Although even the savviest six- or seven-year-old is unlikely to dig into a bowl of the stuff for lunch, cottage cheese does have a reputation as a low-cal food, most often served up alongside a beef patty and fruit cocktail on lunch-counter "diet platters." Cottage cheese only half deserves its reputation. The version made from whole milk, usually labeled *creamed*, has, on average, 117 calories, 5 grams of fat, and 17 milligrams of cholesterol per half-cup serving; nearly 40 percent of its calories come from fat. You'd be better off picking up the low-fat variety next time you shop (known as 1 percent milkfat). Then for every 4 ounces you spoon into lasagna or stuff into a baked potato, you'll be adding only about 82 calories, a little over 1 gram of fat, and 5 grams of cholesterol — quite a savings.

Last, but not least — particularly when it comes to fat and cholesterol tallies — is cream cheese. One healthy *shmear* (about an ounce) of the stuff can add nearly 10 grams of fat (most of it saturated), 100 calories, and 31 milligrams of cholesterol to a virtually fat-free and cholesterol-free bagel. Don't fall prey to the recent advertising campaign that suggests that cream cheese is a healthier spread than butter. It isn't. You'll do little better with "light" cream cheese, trimmed of fat by the addition of such ingredients as low-fat cottage cheese and skim milk: An ounce has 5 grams of fat and 60 calories, which still comes to 75 percent fat.

Because even the lightened-up cream cheeses still aren't nearly as low in fat and cholesterol as would be ideal, you may want to try this viable substitute made from nonfat plain yogurt: Line a colander with cheesecloth and spoon in the yogurt; set the colander over a bowl to catch the liquid, and let the yogurt drain in the refrigerator for at least five hours, or overnight. The yogurt in the colander will be the consistency of softened cream cheese, and you can spread it on a bagel as is, mix it with herbs and stuff it into a baked potato, or stir in a teaspoon of maple syrup to make it a substitute for whipped cream.

While we're on the dairy shelf, let's not forget those gallon jugs full of whole milk. You should already feel like an expert on this beverage. If your kids are under the age of two (in the vital period in which fat and cholesterol are necessary for the full development of brain cells and nerves), go ahead and have them polish off that jug of whole milk, and put skim on your own grocery list. Even 1- and 2-percent milk won't do for yourself or your children older than two. These milks are still fairly high in fat and cholesterol. If your little ones are turned off by the thinner taste and texture of skim, don't take them off whole milk cold turkey. Switch to one of the lower-fat milks until they get used to that; then gradually serve up skim more and more often until they're used to it. Making the transition to healthy eating needn't be a torturous undertaking; helping your children to enjoy the transition will ensure that your changes will have staying power.

Cold cuts, popular for their lunchtime convenience, may be another source of hidden fat and cholesterol, or they may be healthy sandwich makings. Let's start with kids' favorite: bologna. A sandwich-full, about three slices, will supply your child with just over 19 grams of fat—80 percent of the total calories—and 38 milligrams of cholesterol. Salami is only slightly better. Ham, although not perfect, is a slightly healthier deal. Three slices contain 156 calories and 9 grams of fat, which comes out to 52 percent of calories from fat, and 49 milligrams of cholesterol.

If instead of classic cold cuts you stock your meat drawer with thin-sliced turkey, smoked turkey (which has a cured, "hammy" flavor), or even lean roast beef, sandwich meats are one area you won't have to rethink. All of these are a cut above the traditional deli-counter fare in terms of fat and cholesterol content. Turkey — without its skin, of course — derives only 17 percent of its calories from fat; that is, in a standard 3½-ounce serving, which has approximately 150 calories, you'll find only about 3 grams of fat. That's a remarkable difference from, say, the bologna described above.

Let's say you know your kids adore bologna, however, and the last time you shopped you were aware that turkey and chicken are better nutritional bargains. Thinking you could kill two birds with one stone (pardon the poultry pun), you picked up a pack of turkey bologna. You get points for effort, but I'm afraid you really aren't doing any better for your family by bringing such cold cuts home. Here's why: Supposing, for the sake of argument, the particular brand of turkey bologna you bought flaunted a label that said "82 percent fat free," as one popular brand does. It sounds good, but as we'll see in more detail in the next chapter, this label is misleading. For now, let me just point out that one slice of this turkey bologna has 60 calories and 5 grams of fat, which means that 75 percent of the calories comes from fat.

What about meats that don't really qualify as cold cuts — the pork roast in the freezer, the lamb chops marinating for tonight's dinner, the ground beef waiting to be shaped into a meat loaf? No doubt you're aware of meat's heart-harming reputation. The good news is that, although too much meat can send fat, calorie, and cholesterol counts soaring, eaten in moderation and properly prepared, many cuts of meat are perfectly healthy. In fact, meat packs some essential nutrients, including protein, iron, zinc, and the B vitamins.

How can you tell if the meat in your fridge or freezer meets healthy standards? The leanest cuts come from the part of the animal that moves the most (the flank and the shoulder); meat from the more sedentary areas, such as the ribs, are fattiest. I've listed below the leanest cuts of beef, pork, lamb, and veal; these are the ones to shop for.

Beef

Chuck shoulder
Extra-lean ground beef
Eye round
Top round steak
Sirloin tip
Filet mignon
Flank steak

Pork

Tenderloin
Loin chop

Lamb

Shank
Loin chop
Leg

Veal

Cutlet
Shoulder steak
Chop

Besides buying lean, you can prepare and cook meat so that it's as low in fat and cholesterol as possible. For starters, trim away as much visible fat as you can, and then choose a cooking method that requires little, if any, added fat. Rely instead on herbs and vegetables to season meat (like the carrots, onions, and potatoes in a beef stew). The best ways to cook meat are broiling, grilling, and barbecuing; braising and stewing, both of which involve cooking meat for relatively long periods in liquid (broth, wine, or water); and roasting (setting the meat on a rack allows the fat to drip away from the meat).

It's even possible, with patience and perseverance, to lighten up ground meat for use in kid-friendly recipes like spaghetti sauce, enchiladas, lasagna, and chili. The following formula was devised not long ago by a biophysicist from the Boston University School of Medicine. Ironically, it uses oil to help remove the fat, but trust me, it works:

Skinny Ground Meat

2 pounds raw ground beef, veal, pork, or lamb
1½ cups vegetable oil
2 cups boiling water

1. Add the meat to the oil, and heat to 176–194 degrees Fahrenheit while stirring. Use a candy thermometer.
2. Stir for 5 minutes, allowing meat and oil to mix thoroughly.
3. Then, heat to boiling, about 212 degrees Fahrenheit, for 5 more minutes while stirring.
4. Drain through a colander, catching the oil in a bowl.
5. Pour the boiling water over the meat in the colander, collecting the water in the same bowl the oil drained into.
6. Separate the fat from the broth by cooling the container in the refrigerator until the fat hardens on top and can be skimmed off. The now fat-free broth can be added immediately to the cooked meat or boiled first to reduce the volume. Makes about five cups of low-fat chopped meat.

After hamburger come hot dogs, a favorite kid food if there ever was one. The trouble is that one little beef frank consists of about 82 percent fat and contains as many as 42 milligrams of cholesterol. That's one dangerous dog! The now-popular pups made of turkey or chicken, like poultry-based cold cuts, aren't really much healthier than those made from beef. They contain both skin and the fattier dark meat.

Speaking of poultry, let's talk turkey—and chicken, and game hens, and other birds. You probably already know that you can literally peel off most of the fat and cholesterol from poultry by removing the skin. It doesn't matter whether you strip the chicken before or after cooking; either way, you can make a substantial difference. For instance, 3½ ounces of roasted chicken breast has over 10 grams of fat with the skin, and only about 4½ grams without it. (Surprisingly, the cholesterol count barely changes.) Also, keep in mind that the white meat, from the breast and the wing, is leaner than the dark meat found on the thigh and the leg.

Finally, if you have some fresh fillets of flounder, say, or salmon or tuna steaks in the refrigerator, just-bought for tonight's dinner, congratulations. You've chosen one of the smartest entrees around, for a variety of reasons. White-fleshed fish, such as flounder, sole, cod, and snapper, is remarkably low in fat (some types have as few as 2 grams of fat in 3 ounces) and cholesterol. Other types of fish are not as low in fat, but the *kind* of fat they contain may actually help to lower blood cholesterol. Some examples are rainbow trout, salmon, halibut, mackerel, tuna, and sardines. These fish are high in what are known as omega-3 fatty acids, unsaturated fats that have been shown to lower the risk of heart disease by reducing both blood cholesterol and the tendency of blood to clot. Granted, your young ones may be fish-haters — many kids are — but even if you can't get a piece of broiled salmon in them, a sandwich made from water-packed tuna once or twice a week will help them reap the benefits of omega-3. Many shellfish are also replete with omega-3's. The best choices are the ones low in cholesterol, including mussels, oysters, and scallops. Remember, though, that the amount of omega-3 likely to be consumed this way is not of vital importance. Your total fat and saturated-fat intake is still what matters most.

Our next few stops are in the produce bin, the fruit bowl, and wherever else you keep fruits and vegetables. As far as fat and cholesterol go, kids can down these foods to their hearts' content (and for their hearts' sake, as some vegetables have been found to be related to a lowered risk of cardiovascular disease and cancer). Only avocados and coconuts may cause problems. Half a medium avocado has *15 grams of fat*! Because it's a fruit, however, the avocado is cholesterol-free. At any rate, a smidgeon of guacamole on a burrito once in a while won't harm your child's health. As for coconut, you're no doubt already aware of the high saturated-fat content of coconut oil; hopefully, your shelves don't harbor any. If, however, you toss in a handful of flaked coconut when making cookies or other snacks, keep the amount you use—and the frequency with which you make those particular recipes—to a minimum, and you'll be safe.

The only other place you may get in trouble with vegetables is with those frozen in butter or cream sauce. Do you have any of those lurking in your freezer? These ready-made side dishes may have convenience appeal, but the sauces cancel out the vegetables' health value by being fat- and cholesterol-laden. Plain frozen vegetables, on the other hand, are fine. In fact, frozen vegetables are far superior to canned ones, which often contain too much sodium. Some vegetables, such as green beans, even benefit from the big chill. They go from farm to freezer so quickly that there's no time for their nutrients to leach out, which is something that can easily happen to produce left sitting for a week on grocery store shelves.

Let's move on now to the pantry or the drawer where you keep your breads, cereals, pastas, and other grain foods. On their own, virtually all of these foods have zero cholesterol and only a tiny bit of fat, if any. It's hard to get into trouble with a slice of whole wheat toast or a bowlful of spaghetti as long as you're careful about what you put on them. However, as we've seen, one type of food is often healthier than another. Take pasta: From macaroni to rigatoni, nearly all shapes and sizes of noodle are heart-healthy, with the exception of those made with eggs. Use up your egg noodles with a nice, low-fat tomato sauce, and then stick with pastas that have "enriched macaroni" on the label. If you really like the size and shape of the classic egg noodle, you're in luck. At least one manufacturer makes them only from the egg white, so they come out light, fluffy, and better for you.

You can't go wrong with most breads, either. Commercial bakeries have jumped on the fat-free bandwagon and have begun turning out lighter-than-ever loaves, but the truth is, most bread is low-fat by definition. A couple of slices of whole wheat usually has no more than 4 or 5 grams of fat, total. The same goes for sandwich rolls, French or Italian loaves, and English muffins, so if your breadbox holds any of these items, you can breathe easy. On the other hand, croissants (made with layers of butter) and biscuits (often lard- or butter-based) are loaded with fat and cholesterol. The same is true of most store-bought muffins. You are better off baking your own and using vegetable oil or margarine, substituting egg whites for some of the whole eggs, and skipping—or at least skimping on—the nuts. Stud your muffins with berries, raisins, or other dried fruit instead.

Crackers are as healthy or unhealthy as what is in them. Many are made with coconut or palm oil (two highly saturated fats), real butter, or even lard. On the other hand, you can find crackers made of healthier ingredients, so the only way to determine if the crackers you have in stock are the good kind or the bad is to read the package labels carefully. Here's a hint: Melba toast and rice cakes are sure winners and can serve as a base for a slice of low-fat cheese or a smidgen of peanut butter as well as any fat-filled cracker.

Something near and dear to almost any child's heart is cereal. At their best, cereals are low-fat, low-cholesterol, nutritious morning meals; at their worst, a serving of cereal is no more than a bowl full of sugar and fat. Unfortunately, many of the cereals marketed for kids fall into the sugar-laden category, so parents may have to stand firm when youngsters beg for the latest TV-hero-shaped cereal.

Ironically, many cereals claiming to be superhealthy really aren't, such as those made from oat bran, which as you may recall, has been touted as a cholesterol-lowering food. The truth of the matter is that, despite some outrageous claims, the extent of the cholesterol-lowering value of oat bran is yet to be fully proven. The evidence is mildly positive at the present time.

What may be harmful, however, are cereals loaded with nuts, which are replete with both fat and cholesterol. Be wary of granola, as well, which is notoriously high in fat (45 percent) and cholesterol (70 milligrams).

The best cereals are the simplest: bran or wheat flakes, rice puffs, oatmeal, and so forth. They have no added sugars or fats and can be sweetened up with fresh fruit.

While we're in the cereal cupboard, let's check around for other morning foods. I'm picking on breakfast because it's the meal that's most likely to get people in trouble. Think about it: You have three or more people on varying time schedules trying to get up and out of the house each morning. A sit-down banquet of carefully, healthfully prepared-from-scratch dishes is impossible for most modern families. Food manufacturers have picked up on the need for quick morning food. Unfortunately, most speedy breakfasts don't make the health grade. Look at the ingredients breakdown of microwaveable breakfasts, for instance, and you'll see that some derive as much as 73 percent of their calories from fat.

It isn't impossible to get a healthy quick meal in the morning, however. The trick is to retain as much control over what goes on your family's plates (or styrofoam trays) as you can. Choose microwave meals that are based on pancakes or waffles; then dress them up with fresh fruit or even jam, rather than butter and syrup. Skip entrees that include bacon or sausage; there's nothing you can do to skim them of fat. Also, steer clear of another popular speedy breakfast item: the doughnut. Deep-fried food dunked in sugar does not make for a healthy meal. Believe it or not, we're in the final stretch of our kitchen audit. Let's take a look at the cooking and other oils you have in your kitchen; then we'll do a snack search to see if the treats you offer your children between and after meals are up to snuff.

You can judge cooking fats by their cover — sort of. What I mean is that you can tell just by looking at the fats you use whether they're heart-healthy or not. You know that saturated fats are the ones that are most likely to boost blood cholesterol. These come from animal sources and are solid at room temperature. Examples are lard and butter. Two vegetable fats are also saturated: coconut oil and palm oil. Unsaturated fats are those that are oils at room temperature, and these come in two varieties, both of which are thought to help lower cholesterol: *polyunsaturates* for sure and maybe *monounsaturates*. Vegetable oils contain both saturated and unsaturated fats. Look for those that have the least amount of the former and the most amount of the latter. Rapeseed oil (more commonly known as canola oil) probably has the lowest amount of saturated fat of all the vegetable oils, but corn, safflower, olive, peanut, sunflower, and soybean oils are all pretty close. As we've seen, diet margarines made from these oils are healthier than butter; the same holds true for mayonnaise and salad dressings. One word of caution: Just because unsaturated fats have been found to help reduce cholesterol levels in the blood doesn't mean you can eat them with abandon. They *are fats* and should be figured into the daily calorie count as such. The important thing is that, of all the fatty foods out there, these are the ones least likely to get you into cholesterol trouble.

Last, but by no means least, we need to evaluate the snacks you have around the house. Let's go back to your freezer for a moment. A quick glance inside should tell you if you're giving your children their just desserts when it comes to frozen treats. Premium ice creams get their rich flavor and texture from a high percentage of milkfat; one popular brand has nearly 18 grams of fat—nearly 75 percent of it saturated—and 51 milligrams of cholesterol. (These numbers refer to 4 ounces of vanilla ice cream.) You're doing better if you've opted for ice milk. Four ounces of vanilla has only 3 grams of fat and 4 milligrams of cholesterol—quite a saving. Frozen yogurt can be a healthy choice, depending on the brand, but only if it is *low-fat* yogurt. Others are as rich in fat, calories, and cholesterol as ice cream, so reading labels is imperative.

The best cold treats are frozen fruit bars; if you keep these around, give yourself a hand. Most varieties are made of pure fruit and/or fruit juice, are low in calories, and have virtually no fat or cholesterol.

Other snack foods are so numerous and varied it would be impossible to cover each and every one, but there are some rules of thumb that can help you evaluate what turns up in your cookie jar or wherever else you store treats. Cookies that are chocolate-based, nut-studded, or cream-filled are probably high in fat and cholesterol. Better picks would be fruit-filled sandwich cookies, such as fig newtons; graham crackers; vanilla wafers; or ginger snaps.

In the candy department, avoid those with lots of chocolate (Peppermint Patties are lower in fat than M & M's, for instance); jelly beans, which have no fat, are one of the best sweets around.

If your family prefers salty, crunchy snacks, you may have a bag of potato or corn chips, cheese puffs, or the like just waiting to be devoured while you're watching the Saturday night movie. Beware: These are all deep-fried, which might be OK if you could eat just one. But who can? Bring out the air-popped popcorn, light microwave popcorn, or pretzels (they're baked) instead.

And there you have it, a complete rundown of the possible heart hazards in your kitchen, as well as ways either to make them healthier or to substitute foods that are healthier but just as tasty. Now, if you found that your kitchen was a fat and cholesterol disaster area, you're going to want to be prepared to do some savvy the next time you hit the supermarket. The next chapter will prepare you for that trip.

6

Supermarket Savvy

The next trip you make down the aisle could be the second most important one in your life (assuming you're married). The aisle I'm referring to is the first one you hit in your grocery store, and the reason it's crucial is that it will mark the start of a lifetime of healthy food shopping. You now know what to feed your kids to keep their weight and their cholesterol levels in check, you know what *not* to feed them, and you're aware of which cooking techniques will only add fat to foods and which methods will maintain food's healthy integrity. And if your kitchen audit left your cupboards bare, you're going to need to get to the store — fast.

Savvy food shopping starts before you even leave the house. Make a list and check it twice. The reasoning is simple. Knowing beforehand what you want to buy will save time; after all, the average grocery store stocks about 25,000 items. More important, if you have down on paper exactly which healthy foods you need to pick up, you'll be less likely to succumb to impulse buying, which is dangerous because you could easily fall for foods high in fat and cholesterol. If you coupon-shop, don't be tempted to clip coupons for junk food just because they offer a great deal. The cents you save will not be worth shortchanging your family's health. Save money instead by buying the produce, fish, low-fat meats, and grain products that your store has on sale.

When you enter the store, list in hand and game plan in mind, keep these two important points in mind:

1. Read labels.
2. Don't believe everything you read.

If that sounds like contradictory advice, never fear. There is a fine art to reading package labels, and thanks to a long-overdue set of regulations issued by the Food and Drug Administration (FDA) in conjunction with the U.S. Department of Agriculture (USDA), that task should become much less confusing than it was even a year ago. The new rules are designed to prod food manufacturers into being more honest and precise about what really goes into their products. Not only will there be standardized definitions for front-of-the-package claims about foods being "light" or "low-fat" or "low-cholesterol," but every packaged item will bear a comprehensive nutritional checklist, including total calories, calories derived from fat, total fat, saturated fat, cholesterol, total carbohydrates, complex carbohydrates, sugars, dietary fiber, protein, sodium, vitamins A and C, calcium, and iron. Each category will be listed "per serving," and serving sizes will be standardized.

Food companies had until early May 1993 to comply; although many no doubt did so long before then, shoppers may still have to interpret the labels currently being used. Although much of the current packaging information is misleading, most food manufacturers do provide a nutritional breakdown of their products. (You can write to a company and ask for the information if it is not printed on the package; food labels must, by law, include the name and address of the manufacturer, packer, or distributor.)

ANATOMY OF A LABEL

The recent health-consciousness-raising has spurred food makers to prey on consumer's concerns about nutrition and its connection to wellness and longevity. We will focus here on cholesterol because not as many product claims pertain to sodium, preservatives, organic foods, sugar, and such.

Nowhere is misleading information more apparent than on the front of food packages, which often proclaim that the tasty morsels inside are "lean," "light" or "lite," "low-cholesterol" or "high-fiber," "low-fat" or "nonfat." I mentioned earlier that the proposed food label guidelines contain standardized definitions for these catch phrases, and with good reason. As it stands now, many of them may mean just about anything; at present, the Food and Drug Administration (sometimes along with the U.S. Department of Agriculture, which regulates meat and poultry products) defines only a few of the labels commonly found on foods. I've listed these below, along with their "official" definitions:

- *Low-calorie*—fewer than 40 calories per serving (or 0.4 calories per gram).
- *Reduced calorie*—at least one-third fewer calories than the "regular" version of the particular product.
- *Fat-free*—less than half a gram of fat per serving.
- *Low-cholesterol*—less than 20 milligrams of cholesterol per serving.
- *Cholesterol-free*—less than 2 milligrams of cholesterol per serving.
- *Light*—means nothing specific; read the label. (The exception is when this term refers to processed meats; "light" bologna, for instance, must contain 25 percent less fat than standard bologna.)
- *Lite*—ditto.

Some food labels try to do your thinking for you by making claims about the health implications of certain ingredients. For instance, you may come across a package of frozen muffins that bears the banner: "Made with oat bran, which helps reduce cholesterol." Right now, food makers often get away with such messages, whether they're based on scientific truth or not. When the FDA gets its way, only labels linking sodium with heart disease, fat with heart disease and cancer, and calcium with osteoporosis (the brittle-bone disease) will be permitted.

So, if you can't trust the front of the label, what *can* you trust? The back, to a certain extent. On labels that list ingredients and provide a nutritional analysis, there is usually enough information for any savvy shopper to figure out just how healthy that particular food is. Again, it's going to get easier, but until that time, here's how to sum up the back of a food label.

There are three important things to look at in terms of fat and cholesterol, whether on a carton of milk, a package of bologna, or a box of "lite" cookies:

- The total number of calories per portion
- The fat content
- The number of milligrams of cholesterol

The number of milligrams of cholesterol per serving is usually spelled out for you right on the label, as is the total number of calories. You can use the latter number to calculate the percentage of calories from fat. It's easy to do, even though the manufacturers don't always help. Food contents are often expressed in both ounces and grams on the same label (a deliberate attempt to confuse consumers? You tell me). It's not necessary for you to know that there are about 30 grams (specifically 28.35) in an ounce. The only bit of nutritional trivia you need to commit to memory is this: Fat has 9 calories per gram. Engrave this in your mind. You can use that one fact to calculate the percentage of fat in any given food. For instance, if the label on a cereal box says there are 100 calories per portion, and that there are 2 grams of fat per portion, simply multiple 2 grams of fat times 9 (the number of calories in a gram of fat), and you'll get 18. That means that the ratio of fat calories to total calories per serving is 18 to 100. Divide 18 by 100 and then multiply by 100 to convert to a percentage: One serving of our fictitious cereal is 18 percent fat.

Let's try a slightly more complicated example: whole milk. An 8-ounce glass of the stuff packs 150 calories and 8 grams of fat. Get our your calculator and figure along: 8 grams of fat times 9 equals 72 calories. That's a ratio of 72 to 150. Divide 150 into 72, multiply by 100, and you get 48. That's right, whole milk is 48 percent fat! See why I don't believe that milk is necessarily the "perfect food" — at least not for kids over two?

I can drive that point home even further by showing you how to figure out how much of a food's calories comes from saturated fat. Remember, there are three kinds of fat: poly-unsaturated, monounsaturated, and saturated. In milk there are 5 grams of *saturated* fat per 8-ounce serving. Let's work that out: 5 grams times 9 equals 45. That's 45 calories of saturated fat, out of a total calorie count of 150 (45/150). Divide 45 by 150, multiply by 100, and you get 30 percent. In other words, one glass of milk contains a whopping 30 percent of saturated fat.

You may be thinking a parent would have to be a mathematical genius to get through a single shopping expedition. That's not so. Take along your calculator, and remember that it will take only a few trips for you to figure out which foods you'll be buying routinely and which you'll be bypassing.

Besides numbers, pay attention to words. Learn how to interpret ingredients listings. The individual items in a food are listed in descending order of quantity, so you can tell if, say, a jar of strawberry preserves has more sugar than berries. Likewise, if fat is listed near the beginning, chances are that the food has quite a bit of it. If a pancake mix claims to contain cholesterol-fighting oat bran, but oat bran is listed third to last in a long line of other ingredients, think twice about whether those flapjacks are really as health-worthy as they claim.

The fats used in foods can be particularly tricky. Manufacturers are allowed to use this kind of wishy-washy phrasing: "May contain one or more of the following . . ." and then they continue to list several different oils or fats. Among those included may be "good" fats (monounsaturated or polyunsaturated) and "bad" fats (saturated). This ambiguity is allowed so that food companies can change the oils they use according to supply and availability; that's all well and good, but it doesn't help the concerned parent to make an informed buying decision. (Steer clear of foods that don't specify which oils they contain.)

You may be wondering which fats are good and which are bad. Here's a partial list:

Good fats	Bad fats
Canola oil	Lard
Safflower oil	Palm-kernel oil
Sunflower oil	Palm oil
Corn oil	Coconut oil
Peanut oil	Cocoa butter
Soybean oil	Hydrogenated oil
Olive oil	Butter
Cottonseed oil	Shortening

Note that a food may contain many of the "bad" fats listed (those of vegetable origin) and still truthfully claim to be cholesterol-free.

Now let's put into practice what we've learned about reading between the lines of food labels. We're going to take a trip through a typical grocery store so that you can become familiar with the healthy offerings. Some of the suggestions we make are a repetition of our recommendations in Chapter 3, but we would rather reiterate our guidelines than have you end up in the checkout line with a shopping basket full of high-fat foods.

ONE AISLE AT A TIME

Chances are that the first area you'll hit in the typical supermarket is the produce section, chock full of fresh fruits and vegetables in all their no-fat, no-cholesterol glory. Choose freely from this section, avoiding coconuts and being frugal about the avocado (both of which are high in fat).

Up ahead is the meat counter. If your instincts tell you to steer clear, guess again. Even some types of red meat are comparable to poultry when it comes to cholesterol, and although beef, pork, and lamb do have more saturated fat than chicken or turkey, you can still afford to serve them to your family once in a while. In the previous chapter, I listed the cuts of beef, veal, pork, and lamb that are naturally leaner than others. (Remember, the "skinniest" pieces of meat come from the part of the animal that moves the most.) The very leanest cuts of beef, lamb, and pork have approximately 3 grams of fat and 25 milligrams of cholesterol per ounce of cooked meat. That's not bad. But you can do more to ensure that you will get the healthiest possible meats. First, look at the meat carefully before you buy it. Years ago, homemakers scouted for "marbling," lots of white interspersed among the red in a piece of meat, because the meat was "tastier." That white is fat; these days, the less marbled the meat, the healthier. Meat should be trimmed of the fat around the edges as well. You can do this yourself, of course, but why pay for the fat? If you can't find an adequately trimmed cut, have the butcher prepare one for you.

Next, check the label. A piece of beef, veal, and lamb is graded "prime," "choice," or "good," depending on how much fat it has, prime being the most marbled. Go for the "good." Note that some stores market "good" meat as "select."

Both fresh and processed meats (bacon, bologna, salami, frankfurters, and sausage) may also flaunt labels proclaiming that the product is "lean," "extra-lean," "light," "lite," or "low-fat." When referring to fresh meat, like steak, these claims may be true. Some meat producers do breed animals that are leaner, feed them special diets, and take other measures to produce meat that is lower in fat. (Cholesterol counts vary little, however.) The glitch is this: Although these special meats are leaner, they are also costlier.

On the other hand, ground meat that is labeled "lean" or "extra-lean" may contain up to 22 percent fat by weight, hardly an improvement. If you want to lighten up your ground meat, try the process described in the previous chapter. Ground poultry, provided it has been made without skin, is a tasty alternative to ground beef in dishes such as meat loaf and pasta sauce.

Processed meats that claim to be low in fat usually aren't. Most of them still derive up to 70 percent of their *calories* from fat; manufacturers have merely used turkey, rice, or some other filler to replace some of the beef or pork in these products. It won't hurt to serve up some sausage or bacon with the Sunday waffles *very* occasionally. Better yet, opt for slices of some lean ham, such as Canadian bacon (see Table 13).

Next door to the meat is poultry, and then fish. These are easy. As a rule, chicken, turkey, game hen, and the like are low in *saturated* fat (be sure to remove the skin before eating); the

Table 13. Comparison of Bacon and Canadian Bacon

Food	Calories	Fat	% calories from fat
Bacon (2 strips)	72	6 grams	75
Canadian bacon (2 slices)	86	4 grams	42

white meat is even leaner than the dark. These birds do contain their fair share of cholesterol. Three ounces of white-meat chicken has 85 milligrams of cholesterol, and the same amount of broiled top-round beef has 84 milligrams. But fat matters more than cholesterol. And don't cook your goose even for those holiday celebrations. Geese and ducks, along with processed poultry products (turkey sausage and chicken franks), are high in saturated fat.

Now let's go from the land to the sea. The fish department is health heaven. Although most sea fare is low in saturated fat and cholesterol, avoid most smoked fish and canned sardines. Of course, how many children crave sardines? But they do love tuna. Buy it canned in water rather than oil, and you cut out two-thirds of the fat. Shellfish are even lower in fat than fin fish, but the cholesterol they contain does vary. Two favorites, shrimp and crab, are higher in cholesterol, but you can enjoy all shellfish occasionally. Just don't drown them in butter.

Eat other fish to your heart's content. Your best choices are fillets of flounder, cod, haddock, perch, grouper, snapper, and halibut. Enjoy them for their heart-healthy low fat content, not just for their good omega-3 fatty acids. Please remember, though, that breading and frying them defeat the purpose. Stick with the fish, not the coated sticks.

Now for the deli counter. When buying fare for the kids' lunch boxes, opt for sliced roast beef, turkey, lean ham, pressed meats, and even Canadian bacon — all relatively low in fat.

Prepared side dishes, such as cole slaw and potato salad, are almost always swimming in mayonnaise, the epitome of high-fat, high-cholesterol foods. Instead, choose marinated vegetables and pasta salads tossed with veggies and a light oil-and-vinegar dressing and herbs. Better yet, make your own, substituting for the mayonnaise the plain, nonfat, or low-fat yogurt you'll find on our next stop: the dairy case.

Some labels on this aisle are relatively reliable. If cottage cheese says it's low-fat, for example, it is. Two popular brands of cottage cheese stack up as follows: The regular 4 percent milkfat variety has 120 calories and 5 grams of fat in a half-cup serving; its low-fat counterpart, which is 1 percent milkfat, has a mere 80 calories per half-cup serving, and only 1 gram of fat. You already know how milk fares: skim is skinnier than 1 percent, which is skinnier than 2 percent, which is skinnier than whole. Period. Buttermilk, by the way, is unfortunately named; it contains little cholesterol and is low in both total fat and saturated fat. In recipes, it can really enrich the flavor of pancakes and baked goods. Nonfat and low-fat yogurts are generally exactly what they say they are. When in doubt, read the labels.

Most cheeses, sour creams, and cream cheeses are high in saturated fat and cholesterol. Farmer cheese and Neufchâtel cheese (which is a worthy substitute for cream cheese) are usually healthier alternatives. Mozzarella and parmesan cheeses made from part-skim milk have less fat than other hard cheeses. Luckily, more and more alternatives to these items are being developed all the time. An excellent example is Land O' Lakes reduced-fat sour cream, which has 10 fewer calories than the 30 calories in a tablespoon of regular sour cream; better yet, it is 6 percent fat, as compared to the usual 18 percent. Again, read those labels, calculate your comparisons, and soon you'll know which alternatives meet not only your health standards, but your family's taste-bud standards as well.

Now, in the dairy case, you'll find butter and margarine. A lot of people believe that by buying the latter, they'll be doing their children a big favor. Unfortunately, it isn't quite that simple. Unlike butter, margarines are made from vegetable oils rather than animal fat, so they are cholesterol-free and significantly lower in saturated fat. But they are equal to butter in calories (about 100 per tablespoon) and total fat (around 11 grams per tablespoon). Furthermore, there are umpteen varieties of margarine to choose from. Some are made with something called *trans fatty acids*, added to help harden margarine into a stick form. Scientists have discovered that these acids actually raise blood cholesterol levels. To avoid them, buy soft margarine sold in tubs (if the margarine is whipped, it means it has been fluffed with air, which fills in for some calories and fat). Table 14 should make margarine shopping easier.

Now for the bread and cereal aisle. Don't rush down this runway. Here you'll be able to find fiber-rich food that's low in fat, cholesterol-free, and inexpensive to boot. Pick breads that list whole wheat or whole grain at the top of their nutrition labels. (Wheat flour doesn't count; it's just like white flour.) The cereal you buy should have at least 2 grams of fiber, less than 8

Table 14. Comparison of Margarines

Product	Calories	Fat (grams)	Saturated fat (grams)
Stick margarine	100	11	1–3
Tub margarine	100	11	1–2
Liquid margarine	90	10	1–2
Butter blend	90	10	2–3
Whipped margarine	70	8	1–2
Margarine spread	60	7	1–2
Diet margarine	50	6	1

grams of sugar, and less than 2 grams of fat per serving. Stay away from cereals that say they have nuts or nut clusters. They add fat along with the crunch, such as granola, which is notoriously high in fat.

You can't go wrong with pasta. The magic word when buying it is *macaroni*. Egg-based noodles and such are unavoidably higher in fat and cholesterol. The new egg-yolk-less noodles are a good alternative, however; they are made with only the whites. Other good choices in this section are grains such as rice, barley, and couscous. The *soluble fiber* found in brown rice, oats, and barley (as well as in beans, grapefruit, strawberries, and carrots) helps lower cholesterol by reducing the absorption of dietary fat. What's more, these foods make great bases for sauces and compare favorably with pasta when it comes to nutritional breakdown.

In this aisle, you'll also come across bread items other than sandwich loaves, such as muffins, tortillas, and croissants. They are fat-packed; skip them. Go for corn tortillas on taco night, rather than flour tortillas, which are usually made with lard. And read the muffin labels. Often so-called bran muffins list bran long after sugar and oil and eggs; you'll have to give their labels a good once-over before choosing.

Now we come to canned and jar foods. Canned fruits and vegetables are convenient sources of nutrients and, like their fresh counterparts, have little or no fat or cholesterol. Pick fruits packed in their own juices to avoid the extra calories that syrup adds, and go for *low-sodium* canned vegetables when possible. Also, look for juices labeled "100 percent pure fruit juice," rather than sugar-laden fruit drinks or punches.

Canned fish — tuna and salmon — are fine substitutes when you don't have time for fresh fish; make sure those you buy are packed in water, not oil, however. Canned, chunked poultry makes it easy to throw together chicken or turkey salad for sandwiches.

Soup also comes in cans and can be an easy part of a quick lunch or a lazy Sunday supper. Soups have been under fire for their high sodium content; if this is a concern for you and your family, read the labels. Sodium is high when it is over 140 milligrams per serving. Pass by the cream-based soups, such as chowders, as these are most likely to be high in fat.

We're coming into the home stretch now. How's your shopping cart holding out? You won't be adding much from the aisle coming up: the oil and salad-dressing section. We've already said several times that the cooking oil with the least amount of saturated fat is canola oil. Buy some, and use if for cooking, as well as mixing your own light salad dressings of oil, lemon juice, and herbs. If you don't have time to create a salad dressing, choose carefully from the offerings here. Regular dressings are almost all high in calories, fat, and cholesterol. Opt instead for diet dressings, which generally have fewer than 10 calories per tablespoon.

Most stores stock their mayonnaise in this aisle as well. Mayo is basically egg yolk and oil — you can practically see the fat and cholesterol in the stuff. The new "light" mayonnaises have about half the calories. Size them up by reading the labels. Better yet, perk up your sandwiches with condiments, such as mustard, which will add only a few calories and no fat or cholesterol.

Next stop: packaged products. Grocery stores are full of boxed mixes for just about everything from muffins to rice pilafs to cakes — too many to enumerate. Suffice it to say that this is where your calculator may come in handiest. Read the nutrient listings, evaluate the numbers, and choose the best of the lot.

I will say a few words about some particular items: snacks.

Kids need treats just as much as they need nutritional fare, and that's fine, as long as they get the healthiest between-meal nibbles. Sound impossible? You'd be surprised at how much "fun food" passes the low-fat, low-cholesterol test. The following is a partial list:

Vanilla wafers
Fig bars
Graham crackers
Animal crackers
Angel food cake (one of the best deals around: it has no cholesterol and only a smidgen of fat; pile on the fresh fruit, and let your kids chow down!)
Gingerbread
Air-popped popcorn
Pretzels (whole wheat, low salt if possible)
Gelatin

Some food manufacturers are experimenting with low-fat and low-cholesterol varieties of cakes, cookies, and pastries. The results are mixed, though one company in particular — Entenmann's — has been pretty successful with its line of fat-free, cholesterol-free desserts. For instance, its cinnamon apple coffee cake has a measly 90 calories per slice and, as the label promises, no fat or cholesterol. Tasty, too.

Speaking of snacks, childhood wouldn't be childhood without the ultimate treat: ice cream. The myriad of companies that make frozen desserts have really jumped on the health bandwagon, which becomes obvious as we head up the frozen-foods aisle. Supermarkets offer low-fat varieties of ice cream; all sorts of frozen, low-fat yogurts; frozen fruit bars; and tofu-based items. Technology has permitted ice-milk makers to come out with products that are thicker and richer tasting than the old-fashioned watery ice milks. Some of the frozen yogurts are a good choice, though just because a frozen dessert is made from yogurt does not mean it's low in fat. As a rule of thumb, look for products that have 4 or fewer grams of fat per 4-ounce serving. Some good bets, along with their nutritional profiles, are listed in Table 15.

Along with these temptations you'll find other fare among the frozen foods. As I mentioned earlier, frozen vegetables are often even a healthier choice than fresh, as they hit the ice before there's time for their nutrients to be lost. Skip the butter-sauced or cream-sauced ones. There's a wide array of frozen diet dinners out there as well. In a pinch, they can make nutritious, low-fat, and low-cholesterol meals for youngsters on the go (or for youngsters with parents on the go). Choose those with fewer than 15 grams of fat, 400 calories, and 800 milligrams of sodium.

Table 15. Low-Fat Frozen Desserts

Brand	Calories	Fat	% of calories from fat
American Glacé, Dutch chocolate	73	0	0
Frozfruit and Yogurt bar, strawberry (2.5-oz. bar)	90	0	0
Haagen-Dazs frozen yogurt, chocolate or vanilla	173	4	21
Simple Pleasures, chocolate chip	150	3	18
Steve's Gourmet Free, deep chocolate mousse	133	0	0
Tofutti, Lite Lite strawberry or mocha	90	1	10
Soft Serve			
Haagen-Dazs nonfat frozen yogurt, chocolate	120	<1	<8
McDonald's low-fat yogurt cone, vanilla	100	<1	<9
TCBY nonfat frozen yogurt, vanilla	110	<1	<8

By the way, there are a number of frozen dinners packaged specifically for kids. Some of these are atrociously high in calories, fat, and cholesterol. Just because a dinner looks fun to eat doesn't make it good to eat. On frozen-meal nights, give the kids a boring old grown-up TV dinner, and top it off with one of the treats listed in Table 15.

Let's head for the checkout line; your cart should be brimming with good, good-for-your-family things to eat. If this first trip seemed long and complicated, take it from me: Next time around you'll be able to whiz through the market, a seasoned veteran of healthy supermarket shopping.

7

Fast Food, School Food, Camp Food
Is Any of It Good *Food?*

Most books on cholesterol reduction have a chapter on dining out, which usually includes sensible advice on how to read menus, on whether to order stir-fried chicken or the sweet-and-sour pork in a Chinese restaurant, on the relative merits of various salad dressings, on substituting sherbet for the parfait for dessert, and so forth. All of this is well and good. But as you and I and every other parent know, this information is of little value when it comes to kids. When was the last time you went to a fancy French restaurant with your five-year-old? Do you think the average ten-year-old even knows what coq au vin *is?*

In this chapter we'll talk about what to do when you dine out with your kids — and *dine* is a relative term, I realize — at a kids' kind of place. First and foremost among such places is that great American invention, the fast-food restaurant.

Of course, fast food isn't just kids' food. In fact, every day 20 percent of all Americans can be found in fast-food restaurants, munching their Big Macs, their Whoppers, or Dave

Thomas's latest big burger at Wendy's. It's no wonder that fast food is a $70-billion-a-year industry. And it's no surprise to anyone that the biggest name in fast foods, McDonald's, sells 50 percent of all the hamburgers sold in all the fast-food restaurants put together. In the United States alone, McDonald's serves 250 customers a minute.

What are McDonald's and the other chains serving us? Fast food? Definitely. Junk food? Not necessarily. Fatty food? Yes, indeed — although I'm happy to report that they're changing for the better (and largely as a result of pressure from individuals and consumer groups). Still, consider how fast you can ring up the fat grams in a good, all-American fast-food lunch, say, a quarter-pound cheeseburger, a large serving of fries, and a vanilla shake. The damage is 1,205 calories and 59 grams of fat, equivalent to the entire *daily* allotment for some children.

Is that how you want to use up your child's allotment? Hopefully not. But that doesn't mean you have to scratch fast-food restaurants off the list entirely. Kids love 'em; the prices are right; and they are convenient — after all, they don't call them "fast" for nothing.

In order to make sure that every trip to the local Burger King isn't going to throw off your child's fat allowance for the entire week, we ought to start by separating some myths from facts about fast food. First and foremost is the idea that all fast foods are junk food. As we said earlier, they're not. If you look, you will see some nutritious entrees on the menu. And the situation is getting better. A major sign of progress is that most of the chains now have salad bars. Who would have imagined that twenty years ago?

Yet these signs of progress can be misleading. For example, a baked potato — now a staple at many fast-food restaurants — sounds like a healthy choice, and at 2 grams of fat per plain potato, it is. But that's not how potatoes are usually served in fast-food restaurants. They're stuffed with cheese and, alas, with fat—34 grams of fat to be specific. That's 13 more grams than a quarter-pound hamburger (see Table 16).

And what about those much-ballyhooed "lean" offerings? Well, as we'll see in a moment, although they may be lighter in calories, many have a hefty fat content. Of the 347 calories in a Hardee's Real Lean Deluxe, 35 percent are fat. And Kentucky Fried Chicken's Lite 'n' Crispy skin-free chicken is lighter in weight only. The crispy part is me burning up over the fact that a shocking 50 percent of its calories are fat.

Watch out, too, for those breakfast items. Hardee's new oat-bran muffin sounds heart-healthy (and could appeal mightily to those who believe that oat bran is really some sort of magical cure for high cholesterol), but hold onto your coffee. It has 440 calories and 18 grams (37 percent) of fat.

We applaud Dunkin' Donuts for replacing egg yolks with egg whites. They've done away with cholesterol, but say, guys, could you hold the fat, too? A plain doughnut—breakfast, sad to say, for some kids and adults—is still 37 percent fat (18 grams). Instead, choose Dunkin's "yeast rings." They may have an awful-sounding name, but they're actually lower in fat: A chocolate-frosted yeast ring has only 10 grams.

Finally, much was made of the July 1990 announcements made by McDonald's, Wendy's, and Burger King that they would henceforth cook their fries in 100 percent vegetable oil as

Table 16. *Comparing Quarter Pounders and Potatoes*

Food	Calories	Grams of fat	% Fat
Quarter-pound hamburger	445	21	42
Plain baked potato	250	2	7
Cheese-stuffed potato	590	34	52

opposed to the previous blend of lard and vegetable oil. Good, but before we send bouquets to each, let's remember that a small serving of fries still contains the same amount of *total* fat — about 15 grams, or 135 calories — although it reduces the *saturated* fat.

The fact of the matter is that the fast-food restaurants are not out to "poison America." They are out to make money, and like any good business, they do that by responding to consumer demands. It's fortunate for us that a few consumers have made some healthy demands, most notably Phil Sokolof, an Omaha businessman and "born-again" heart attack victim. Many of the aforementioned changes in the fast-food giants' menus — particularly the change from lard to pure vegetable oil — can probably be attributed directly to the pressure brought to bear by Sokolof's nationwide (and self-financed) advertising campaign, in which he scored the Big Three on their fat-laden foods and preparations. The Committee for the Public Interest also deserves credit for its steady barrage of reports targeting saturated fats as the heart's number one dietary enemy. Thanks to their efforts, as well as to the industry's recognition of our increasing health-consciousness, fast-food restaurants have taken the first steps toward making their menus heart-healthier. But ultimately, they'll stop serving double bacon cheeseburgers and large fries only when we stop ordering them. A McDonald's spokesperson noted that the many "closet cheeseburger eaters" among us, not to mention many "vacillating" consumers, may pay lip service to the idea of healthy eating at home, but they are all too quick to wrap their lips around cheeseburgers and fries when they eat out.

Who's to blame for the fact that fries outsell salads 10 to 1, that Jack-in-the-Box's top seller is its Ultimate Cheeseburger, or that its new Bacon Bacon cheeseburger is a howling success? As Pogo said, "We have met the enemy, and he is us."

There are no statistics documenting how many of those Bacon Bacon nightmares, or comparable fat-laden offerings, are being eaten by children. But even if it's mostly adults who are buying this stuff (and I doubt it), it's safe to say that at least some of them are parents, and they're sending a message to their kids that's terribly, terribly wrong.

Again, that's not to say you can't—or won't—ever go to fast-food restaurants. But when you do, and particularly when you order for and with your children, vote with your heart. This is becoming easier now that these restaurants are beginning to give you some healthier choices. Let's review each fast-food chain, option by option. After spending many hours and a few dollars at each, we've decided to give each of the major fast-food restaurants an arbitrary letter grade based on:

- The availability of nutritional information
- The number and quality of lower fat choices on the menu

McDONALD'S

Before we offer a critique of the industry leader, here is a little background information:

With 11,400 restaurants in fifty-three countries, McDonald's is the largest fast-food chain in the world. When it makes changes, it makes news—as in 1990, when the chain announced that ingredient and nutrition information for its products would be posted in all of its restaurants. McDonald's made headlines again in the spring of 1991, when the company announced the introduction of the McLean burger.

The McLean story is revealing. Developed at Auburn University with the help of a $300,000 grant from the Beef Industry Council, the McLean was touted as a real breakthrough fast-food product. It was a 91 percent fat-free (by weight, we should add) quarter-pound hamburger, made with the seaweed derivative carrageenan and water. The introduction of the product was remarkably fast. Whereas McDonald's has been test-marketing pizza for over five years, for example, McLean went from drawing board to menu board in just nine months. And once it hit the stores, even Phil Sokolof was impressed. He called it "a great day for the American people." Indeed, it was significant if only because it improved on the existing low-fat burgers of the rival chains Wendy's and Hardee's, which were only 10 to 15 percent lower in fat than their regular burgers.

But again, let's read the fine print here. When we convert the expectedly misleading "91 percent fat-free" — which is 9 percent fat by weight — to calories, it suddenly becomes 29 percent fat. Now compare that to the old quarter-pounder, as shown in Table 17.

Although McLean is a step in the right direction, I'm not ready to call McDonald's a health-food restaurant yet, despite the changes it's made in its menu:

- It changed to all-vegetable oil for cooking fries and hash browns.
- It changed from 2 percent to 1 percent low-fat milk.
- It now offers low-fat milkshakes (0.5 percent fat).
- It now offers low-fat yogurt (0.5 percent fat).
- Fat-free fruit sherbet dressings are now available at some outlets.
- It offers whole-grain breakfast cereals and low-fat, no-cholesterol muffins (containing only 480 calories and just 10.5 percent, or 5.6 grams, of fat).
- It reduced salt in the hamburgers, sausage, hotcakes, and pickles.

Table 17. See the Difference in Burgers

	McLean	Regular
Weight (oz.)	7	6
Total calories	310	410
Grams of fat	10	20.7
% fat (as calories)	29	45
Grams of saturated fat and estimate % of fat	4 (11.6%)	8 (17.5%)

Considering the visibility of this franchise — and the extent to which it's ballyhooed its improvements, the poor availability of nutritional information within each of its restaurants is surprising. Many other chains offer a toll-free 800 number for consumers to call. If you want to learn the ingredients of one of McDonald's entrees or to offer feedback on what you've eaten, the call to Illinois comes out of your pocket. And despite the improved entrees we listed, there are some McClinkers. For example, their chicken McNuggets have 56 percent fat, 56 milligrams cholesterol, and 580 milligrams of sodium, and their barbecue sauce, although only 9 percent fat, has 340 milligrams of sodium in only 1 ounce.

Overall, though, I think we should give McDonald's its due. It's not only the biggest fast-food chain, but it seems to be the leader when it comes to making an effort to provide more low-fat alternatives for you and your child. I just hope this effort continues.

BURGER KING

Not to be outdone by its archrival, BK claims to have introduced its own share of lower fat products and also displays its nutritional and ingredient information — although, as we found in most chains, these displays are as perfunctory as fire-inspection and building-occupancy certificates.

If you can't read the fine print on the posted nutrition board at Burger King, you can call 1-800-937-1800. Alas, after doing my research, I was ready to call that number to complain. Look at these average fat percentages for major BK offerings:

- Burgers: 51 percent
- Chicken sandwiches: 48 percent
- Fish sandwich: 45 percent
- Salad dressings: 88 percent
- Average sodium for all sandwiches: 822 milligrams, more than half of what your child should have in an entire day

How about BK's breakfasts? Not much better, I'm afraid. A plain croissant is 50 percent fat, and the average croissant sandwich is 60 percent. Even BK's bagel sandwich turns a usually low-fat item into a 40 percent fat feast. Muffins average 44 percent, and the raisin oat bran weighs in at 37 percent.

It's enough to drive you to drink. But if you do drink, you may want to think twice before drinking milk at BK. It has whole milk at 51.5 percent, and its 2 percent milk (by weight) is actually 37 percent fat (by calories). By contrast, its shakes average 27 percent, thanks to — Would you believe? — low-fat chemicals.

I had to ask myself, "Am I missing something on their nutritional poster?" Was their table bare? I called BK's toll-free number and was given good news. BK was finally getting onboard. In addition to its "nutritional poster," a new "nutritional guide" is now becoming available at some of its restaurants. Produced in collaboration with Weight Watchers, the guide appears under the name, "Your Way, the Lighter Way." The foods are not "lighter" in calories, and certainly not in salt, but they do give you the chance to choose less total fat, less saturated fat, and less cholesterol. Table 18 illustrates the point.

Burger King, like many other restaurants and supermarkets, is increasingly making healthier food choices available. More and more, the ball is in our court.

In terms of its heart-healthy offerings, I think Burger King is second to McDonald's, but gaining ground fast.

Table 18. Burger King Better Buys

	Calories	% total fat	% saturated fat	Cholesterol (milligrams)	Sodium (milligrams)
BK broiler	267	27	7	45	728
Fettucini broiled chicken	298	33	12	75	840
Angel hair pasta, no cheese	160	11	N/A	5	170
Angel hair pasta, with cheese	210	21	4	10	330
Broiled chicken salad	140	26	6	39	440
Veggie sticks	60	15	0	0	75
Tropicana fruit twister	50	0	0	0	28
Mocha pie	160	28	16	5	150
Chocolate frozen yogurt	132	21	14	10	40
Chocolate brownie	100	27	Less than 9	5	150
Creamy ranch salad	35	0	0	3	140

WENDY'S

Wendy's has no 800 number and seems to follow the industry standard of posting information closer to the parking lot than to the serving line.

As for its offerings, Wendy's is better than BK in the most popular items. Its burgers average 43 percent fat, and chicken is 37 percent. Again, though, don't get hooked by fast-food fish sandwiches. They're more foul than fish, weighing in at 49 percent fat. There's also a steak sandwich at Wendy's that adds up to 51 percent fat.

Wendy's was one of the first major fast-food chains to promote prepared salads. It currently has three—chef's, garden, and taco—with an average fat content of 33 percent. That's not too bad, but you should choose carefully at the salad bar, where, the dressings average 90 percent fat. We also salute Wendy's for offering a simple baked potato, one of the few items offered by any fast-food chain that has almost *no* fat. But if you let your child have one of the varieties stuffed with cheese, sour cream, and so on, you haven't done her or him any favor. The fat content of these treats jumps to anywhere from 34 percent to 52 percent.

Wendy's two desserts average 34 percent fat as well, and you can wash them down with chocolate milk—28 percent fat—or worse yet, with Wendy's "2 percent" milk, which is actually 33 percent fat by calories.

KENTUCKY FRIED CHICKEN

The KFC chain faces a major problem: Its entire "finger-lickin' good" reputation is based on the fact that its chicken is fried and heavily coated, so that it is often higher in saturated fat than a hamburger. KFC has tried to deal with this in a couple of ways, first, by simply changing its name to the acronym KFC, and second, by introducing a new fried, skinless chicken entree, which was touted as having fewer calories and less fat, cholesterol, and salt than the "original" recipes.

Why did KFC even bother? On our visit to a local outlet, we found no 800 numbers, no posted information, and no literature. In fact, we saw nothing but fat—in the oil, in the coatings, in the entrees, and even in the advertising for the skinless chicken.

ROY ROGERS

No 800 numbers here—not even a professionally produced nutrition posting. The one we saw was filled with glaring errors (such as listing milligrams of fat instead of grams) and was very difficult to read.

As far as health and cholesterol for your child are concerned, Roy Rogers doesn't even *offer* a low-fat burger, and his regular burgers average 49 percent fat. Chicken parts are a whopping 56 percent, and the fish sandwich is predictably high at 42 percent. Average sodium at Roy's? 758 milligrams per sandwich. Now, Roy's roast beef sandwiches average 32 percent and is a wise choice for consumers.

Roy's salads tempt fate with six of the most popular choices averaging 54 percent fat (chopped eggs, granola, macaroni salad, potato salad, cole slaw, and Greek pasta). The salad dressings average 85 percent, none are low-fat, and even the "low-calorie Italian dressing" is 77 percent fat.

HARDEE'S

Hardee's not only has an 800 number (1-800-346-2243), but it has some lovely people at the other end of the line in Rocky Point, North Carolina, who provide Hardee's nutritional information to us with a side dish of southern charm.

The chain's burgers, though, are nothing to call home about, with an average fat content of 50 percent, and the lone fish entree is 43 percent fat. But the roast beef sandwiches average a satisfactory 32 percent (the same as those at Roy Rogers), and at only 29 percent fat, the chicken sandwiches are the healthiest of those at any of the six chains we investigated. (Watch out for the chicken pieces, though, which average 40 percent.)

The chicken and pasta salad here is another fine fast-food choice, averaging a terrific 12 percent fat, but choose wisely: The chef's salad has over four times the amount of fat, averaging 56 percent.

Breakfasts offer a similarly wide range: 6 percent fat for three pancakes is a great nutritional deal, but if you add bacon or sausage, all bets are off at 29 percent. Steer your children away from the "Big Country" breakfast; it's 52 percent fat. Instead, get them the pancakes, a delicious and nutritious enough breakfast for any country, big or small. With margarine, the pancakes are still only 12 percent fat.

For dessert, you can enjoy a shake for 17 percent fat or an ice cream cone or sundae for 30 percent, but you can also blow your child's fat budget with the apple turnover (40 percent) or the dreaded "Big Cookie" (47 percent).

At Hardee's, the choices are there, but you have to make them with your eyes wide open.

As we said in the beginning, if you have kids, it's awfully hard to avoid fast-food restaurants. Even if you don't take the kids, they'll end up there anyway as they get older. So, let's get them into the habit of choosing correctly now. Here are some general guidelines to help you along:

- Order burgers without toppings of cheese, bacon, or mayonnaise.
- Skip the fish sandwiches; they may sound lower in fat, but as we've seen, they're not.
- When ordering chicken, choose white meat instead of dark, and choose skinless or original coating instead of crispy.
- Choose the chains with wider selections: salad bars, baked potatoes, and so on. (But be careful at those salad bars: Remember the hidden fats).
- Unless they have a low-fat yogurt or sherbet option, skip desserts at fast-food restaurants. Save the treat for home, where you have more control.
- Order soft drinks or iced tea instead of milkshakes.

Finally, *think* about what you're going to order *before* you go in — or certainly before you get in line. It's virtually impossible to read the posted nutritional information — in order to count your fat grams — without stepping out of line and thereby risking the ire of impatient, foot-tapping folks behind you.

Remember: It may be fast food, but your child's health should never be a rushed decision.

OTHER FAST-FOOD RESTAURANTS

We've focused above on the major hamburger and chicken fast-food chains, but there are other restaurants that serve the kinds of foods that parents and kids love, food that's tasty, inexpensive, and fast. As a parent and pediatrician, I have two come to mind immediately: pizza and Chinese food.

PIZZA

No wonder pizza is a $15-billion-a-year business in the United States. Adults love it. Kids love it. What hooks kids on pizza, I think, is more than the taste. As I'm sure you've found out, kids love to eat with their hands, and pizza enables them to do that without being reprimanded by you — because you're sitting across the table doing the same thing!

Although neatness doesn't count with pizza, nutrition does. Pizza is a fairly nutritious food, and it can be heart-healthy as well, provided you make it that way. How? By ordering it with a tomato base instead of cheese — or at the very least, by asking for low-fat cheese and less of it. If you use toppings, order vegetables or seafood, not pepperoni, sausage, or meatballs. Here's why: One slice with vegetable toppings contains 155 calories and 5 grams of fat (27 percent). One slice with "everything" (which includes pepperoni, sausage, meatballs, you name it) contains 240 calories and 12 grams of fat (45 percent).

Many — perhaps most — local pizzerias now offer such alternative toppings and will accommodate your requests. Surprisingly, at the major pizza chains we contacted — Domino's, Pizza Hut, and Pizzeria Uno — we were told that you take it the way they serve it, which means high in fat. So we recommend taking your business to a place that will give you and your child a chance, and a choice — probably your local, family-run pizzeria.

CHINESE FOOD

For the kids, Chinese food is fun and festive, and looks cool, too. For parents, it's tasty and inexpensive — and usually available quickly. It's long been a family staple in the New York area and, I think, in most other parts of the country as well.

Remember that we said the average cholesterol level among people in rural China is about 150? Well, they didn't get that from eating sweet-and-sour pork, Peking duck, or most of the other banquet foods that are the typical fare of American Chinese restaurants. However, there are lots of healthy choices you can make here.

It's often noted that nobody prepares vegetables the way the Chinese do. I agree, and I think it's a great way to get your kids to start enjoying vegetables, too. So don't be afraid to choose a "Buddhist delight," or just a shrimp with broccoli or chicken and mixed vegetables.

Avoid the fried rice and go for lo mein, instead. For the uninitiated, lo mein is Chinese pasta. Or to be more historically accurate, pasta is Italian lo mein. Avoid egg rolls; spring or shrimp rolls are lighter. Of course, duck the duck, and skimp on the sauces. Most Chinese restaurants no longer put MSG on their foods, and many will use lighter sauces if requested. Soy sauce has no fat at all, but it's loaded with salt: 1,029 milligrams per tablespoon, which is two-thirds of your child's daily salt allotment.

Wonton soup is fine — the average fat content is only 20 percent — but drop the eggdrop and can the Cantonese. For dessert, bypass the ice cream, order fruit, and let your child have a fortune cookie — if you're following the advice in this book, we predict a lower cholesterol level in the very near future.

SCHOOL LUNCHES

To some people, every big problem in our society is the fault of big government. Of course, that's not always true, but in the case of nutrition, poor school lunches and the miserable eating habits they've helped to instill in our children do indeed place a large part of the blame on one big department in our government: the U.S. Department of Agriculture (USDA). You have to hand it to the folks at the USDA. Once they've got their mind set on an idea, not even several decades of scientific research or the consensus of most nutritionists will change it.

The four food groups are our case in point. The USDA, which is responsible for distributing surplus foods to schools, adopted this approach to diet and menu planning almost half a century ago, and until recently, they were still beating the same old drum, even though it was out of step with everything that modern nutritional science is telling us.

As we've noted, the USDA's emphasis on red meat, eggs, and whole milk is probably part of the reason this country has high cholesterol levels in the first place. Generations of meat-, egg-, and milk-consuming Americans grew up learning about the four food groups from USDA posters, pamphlets, and films, and it seems that some people at the department itself still believe their own propaganda. As recently as 1989, a USDA spokesperson assured us that "There are no good or bad foods. As long as you eat a variety of foods in moderation, that's the way to go." The result? School lunches with an emphasis on milk, butter, eggs, and ground beef—great for the dairy and meat industries, but not so great for our kids.

Fortunately, as in the fast-food industry, things are getting better. School and camp lunches, long the butt of jokes, are improving without—or is it despite?—the help of organizations like the USDA or the beef and dairy lobbies. The credit for improved institutional meals belongs partially to local school and camp dieticians, most of whom seem to be making an honest effort to improve the nutritional value of the food offered.

The improvement is also due to parents like you. The impetus for change sometimes comes from outside the school.

That translates into parents taking an interest and getting involved, either as individuals or through the PTA — the main function of which, one local PTA president reminded us, is to be an advocate for the children.

This same woman's PTA recently demonstrated not only its concern but its power when, in response to complaints about the quality of the food and the conditions at a local school cafeteria, it formed a committee of parents who went in and observed the operation. They made recommendations to the school administration, which were accepted. Changes were made, and in at least one school, the kids are eating better now.

Advocating a healthy, low-fat diet in the schools is something that should be on the agenda of every PTA. To make sure a healthy menu is being served to your child, start by looking at the school menus that will be mailed to you, or that your child will bring home. If you don't like what you see, call the school or your local PTA, and get some answers to questions like these:

- Is the food prepared on the site or nearby?
- Is there a registered dietician on the staff?
- Is the cafeteria clean and attractive? Are there efforts to promote healthy eating — or is the cafeteria posting the same, old USDA posters showing smiling kids eating a "healthy" breakfast of bacon, eggs, and milk?
- Is salad offered, including beans and low-fat cheeses?
- Are skim, 1 percent, and chocolate skimmed milk available?
- Are 100 percent fruit juices available?
- Is there a good selection of fresh fruits and vegetables?
- Are whole-grain breads available? Is there margarine instead of butter?
- Are any luncheon meats low-fat or low-salt?

- Is poultry or fish available, and is it prepared and served without breading?
- Are turkey dogs offered as substitutes for beef or pork?
- Are low-fat yogurt and low-fat frozen yogurt available?
- Are foods routinely fried, or are broiled and baked entrees regularly served as well?
- Are cookies made without palm or coconut oil? Good cookies are oatmeal-applesauce, pumpkin-raisin, or fig-filled, and remember that angel food cake is one of the most low-fat, high-taste desserts you can serve.

A popular alternative to buying lunch is, of course, bringing your lunch from home, typically a sandwich. Here again, though, we have to be careful about what we stick between those two pieces of bread. To make a smarter, healthier sandwich for your child, use whole-grain breads and limit the spreads. Substitute low-fat seasoned yogurt for some of the mayonnaise; use low-fat cottage cheese to stretch fillings; and throw in some chopped vegetables, sprouts, or sunflower seeds for flavor—and nutrition.

And let's not get caught in a BLT or bologna rut. Here are some healthy sandwich suggestions:

Bread	Filling
Whole wheat	Tuna salad (add vegetables and sunflower seeds)
Pita	Low-fat cottage cheese and vegetables
Pumpernickel	Low-fat (cottage?) cheese and sliced tomatoes
Italian or French	Sliced turkey or chicken breast
Flour tortilla	Lean beef and sliced peppers
Bagel	Monterey jack, avocado, and salsa

CAMP CHOW

Every May and June, like most pediatricians, I am up to my ears doing camp checkups. That is the time I get my most reliable feedback about what is going on with camp food—from the children themselves. When I talk to the camp directors or their representatives, their reassurances about their food are as glowing as the camp brochures and videos we have all seen. Their descriptions of the menus appear to have been taken right out of a nutritionist's "how-to" guidebook. The reality, though, is usually (but not always) a bit different.

When I asked twelve-year-old Lee, a representative camper, what the food had been like at his camp the previous year, he responded innocently, "Normal stuff, like hamburgers, hot dogs, and grilled-cheese sandwiches." Getting down to specifics, breakfast meant choosing from boxes of dry cereals, waffles, pancakes drenched in syrup and butter, French toast, cream cheese, and eggs. There was a choice of whole or skimmed milk, and you could have juice. Lunch was cold cuts, usually bologna, salami, or maybe sliced turkey, as well as bread and butter, macaroni and cheese, and the ubiquitous peanut butter. Dinner was—you guessed it—hamburger, hot dogs, meat loaf, or roast beef. Fish? What's that? My hat is off to some camps that now offer a salad bar at lunch and dinner.

Granted, as one mother told me when we talked about camp fare, "It's only two to eight weeks out of the year." But remember that one of our goals is to improve the long-term eating habits of our children, including when they are out of their parents' watchful sight.

My suggestion is to ask the camp representatives judicious questions. Ask them to get away from the "party line" and level with you. I have found this to be a sound tactic. You do not expect Camp Pritikin, but you have a right to expect to have sensible alternatives to "normal" camp food available so that your child at least has choices. Whether or not he or she makes good choices depends on what you are able to accomplish in the other forty-four to fifty weeks of the year.

SNACKING AT THE SHOPPING MALL

Snacking is not just a convenience; it's a necessity. Kids need to snack because they have smaller stomachs and higher energy levels. So after being dragged around a mall for a few hours, they're going to get very hungry, no matter what time of day it is.

Contrary to popular belief, you can eat well in a mall, or in a theater, or at the zoo, or in any other public place where the choices might seem to be between a hot dog or a wad of cotton candy. As is the case anywhere else — school, fast-food restaurants, and your supermarket — there are better choices that can and should be made.

In the case of typical mall food, there are many unhealthy choices that you should definitely avoid. Consider the fat content of some of these kiosk staples:

- Hot dog with mustard: 240 calories and 14 grams of fat (52 percent fat calories)
- Soft pretzel with cheese: 275 calories and 8 grams of fat (26 percent)
- Quarter-cup of mixed nuts: 225 calories and 21 grams of fat (84 percent)
- Large chocolate-chip cookie: 190 calories and 8 grams of fat (38 percent)
- Ice cream cone, single scoop: 190 calories and 9 grams of fat (43 percent)

But remember, not all snack foods are junk foods, and you can transform even some of the "junky" things we've just mentioned into low-fat, healthy foods simply by ordering right, thinking twice, and making an intelligent substitution or two. For example, the soft pretzel with cheese is a killer. Hold the cheese, please, and you have a snack that's almost fat-free. It's the same thing with popcorn. Hot butter equals heavy fat; there are 8 grams (69 percent fat calories) in the cup of popcorn sold at your typical movie theater concession stand. Ask for it without butter, and, presto, you've got a snack that's nutritious, filling, tasty, and practically fat-free. Finally, you can steer your child away from ice cream and direct her or him toward a cool, luscious cup of low-fat frozen yogurt. You will have saved about 8 grams of fat from your daily allotment.

In summary, the principles in choosing what to eat are the same wherever we eat. They get back to choosing wisely and keeping the big picture in mind. We can still balance out the occasional splurge and the inevitable weak moment (either your child's or your own) with more healthy selections later that day or the next day. Or you can let your child burn off some of these calories with exercise—the other part of the cholesterol-reducing equation, which we'll address in the next chapter.

8

Child's Play

The Other Side of the Cholesterol Equation

Not long ago, we visited a midtown Manhattan health club at lunchtime and watched as a contingent of middle-aged corporate execs, lawyers, and Wall Street big shots — some of them younger than I — walked the treadmills and pedaled away on the stationary bikes. Young physiologists with clipboards in hand carefully monitored their pulses as they huffed and puffed along.

Those exercising looked so grim — even a bit scared. And with good reason. Many of these men had suffered heart attacks or some other heart-related problem. They had been referred to this club by their cardiologists, who know that a moderate exercise program will help strengthen the cardiovascular system, reduce body fat, and hopefully prolong life.

I was glad to see that these men were following their doctors' advice. However, I couldn't help thinking what a shame it was that they had waited this long. It took nothing less than a brush with death to get them out of their chairs and onto their feet. They had paid the price for a lifetime of neglect. Didn't they wish that they had started on the right path years ago?

Your child can. Although the focus of most of this book has been on diet, exercise is an increasingly important factor in the cholesterol-reducing equation. Although the evidence here is not yet as conclusive as it is on the benefits of a low-fat diet, new studies are being published all the time. Studies have found that exercise can increase the beneficial HDLs and lower blood pressure and is a good way to reduce obesity in children, which is a major problem in this country and one that I'm convinced is linked, in many cases, to high cholesterol levels in later life. Show me an overweight child, and I'll show you a sedentary, overweight adult with high cholesterol levels and a high risk of heart problems. Lean, active kids, on the other hand, tend to grow into lean, active athletic adults, who are more likely to have sound diets, higher HDLs, and substantially lower odds of suffering from heart disease.

So if you're concerned about your children's cholesterol levels or, indeed, about their overall health, it's high time to get them on an exercise program. Obviously, we can't provide you with all of the information you might need in one chapter. However, we can share with you some of the insights and ideas of people I respect, starting with the man who is widely credited with starting the exercise boom in America for adults: Dr. Kenneth Cooper.

It's not surprising that Cooper is a big advocate of controlling cholesterol in children through exercise. A cardiologist, he is best known as the author of *Aerobics*, the 1968 best-seller that introduced Americans to this form of exercise. Cooper recommends that you get your child actively involved in vigorous play and walking at the earliest ages, but he's careful to point out that youngsters should not begin long-distance, structured aerobics until the age of ten. "I become concerned when parents start their children running for miles at a very young age," he wrote.

So do I — and it's not only running long distances but lifting weights that I'm concerned about. I recommend neither for any child under twelve, and not just because such stressful activities may cause problems in still-developing muscles and bones. There's something more fundamental: If we want kids to exercise, we have to make it fun. The last thing I'd want to see a child doing is the kind of structured, regimented program followed by adults in a health club. Why? Try to get your child to sit on a stationary bike for thirty minutes. I suspect this exercise program will probably last for a grand total of about ten minutes. By comparison, let me tell you about another club I visited in another part of New York City.

I had been asked to advise on an exercise program for thirteen-year-old Benjamin, a young man from the projects. Ben lived in a neighborhood so tough that his mother was afraid to let him outside after school. Not surprisingly, he began spending more and more time in front of the TV. But Benjamin was lucky. He was selected by a local newspaper to be part of a story in which sedentary individuals were matched up with personal trainers, and their progress was followed over time. With his mom's enthusiastic support, Benjamin was matched up with Lesley Howes, the owner of a trendy aerobics studio in SoHo. Lesley, who grew up outside Toronto in a sports-minded family, jumped at the opportunity. "It's been my dream to work with kids ever since I moved to New York," she said. "I'm amazed at how totally out of shape American kids are."

I'm not, of course. I see them in my office every day. It's estimated that one in every four schoolchildren in this country is overweight. That's consistent with my observation — and what's more disturbing is that it seems to be getting worse. The numbers of obese children in our practice have almost doubled since we started.

How do we deal with this growing problem? Lesley, for one, approaches it from an interesting perspective. "Kids have to learn to be more sensitive and in touch with their own bodies," she said. "They're not going to get that from watching a video game." Nor, I'm afraid, from the kind of structured exercise programs that are followed in most physical education classes. Those have their place, and obviously, the people who teach them contend with serious limitations in time and facilities. But I think these programs can sometimes discourage kids as much as encourage them. "Most phys. ed. programs are based on competition," says Vic Dante, an exercise physiologist and consultant to the New York City Board of Education. "And a lot of kids don't have competitive natures or confidence in their abilities." This, in turn, leads to a failure cycle. The child who feels unable to perform as well as his or her peers will avoid all sports. And because this child probably associates all physical activities with sports, he or she will eventually avoid all sports and fitness-related activities, even though the two are mutually exclusive.

It doesn't have to be that way. By separating exercise from sports — or at least competitive sports — and by making it fun, not something you have to be good at, we can get our kids into the exercise habit. Watching the routine Lesley developed for Ben really opened my eyes to the creative possibilities of noncompetitive exercise for children. She started Ben shadow-boxing. At first, I was a bit concerned. Is boxing the kind of activity we want to promote in kids? But in her workout, there was none of the savagery of pugilism, and all of its grace and balance. Lesley had Ben follow her every move and every swing; I watched the boy grin as he shadow-danced with her across the floor of the studio, getting more nimble and sure of himself with every combination of "punches" he threw and every step he took.

"OK," she cried. "Now I want twenty-five straight-out jabs." I saw Ben's face redden as he began to exert himself. Then he smiled again, as Lesley—a superb athlete—backpedaled across the studio. "Come on, catch me!" she said. Off Ben went, trying to keep stride for stride with Lesley, as she moved fluidly across the room. They stopped while she encouraged Ben to take some water, and then it was on to rope-jumping, the most low-tech kind of exercise you can imagine. "I don't know," said Ben sheepishly when Lesley handed him the rope. "My sister does this, and I'm not very good at it."

Lesley proved you don't need a computerized stair climber to get a good workout. All of the things she did with Ben could be done in his apartment, with a playmate, and for almost no cost. Jumping rope—a time-honored approach to both play and exercise—is a perfect example. Ben started out getting tangled up, but after a while, he was able to jump for three minutes straight, and he told us that he was determined to work at it, in order to get better.

Before I could catch my breath, Lesley and Ben were on to their next "exercise." This one was a game in which Lesley rolled a rubber ball to Ben's left or right, and he had to scramble laterally to get it and roll it back with his hands. Soon, there were two balls rolling simultaneously, and Ben was gliding back and forth like a shortstop during batting practice. He giggled with delight, Lesley laughed, and I couldn't help but smile. Ben was getting a great workout, and just as important, he was having fun, because Lesley had made it seem like a game. And that's the key. As I tell parents, the best activity for your child is the one your child likes best.

I recognize we can't all have personal trainers like Lesley working out with our kids. But more and more people like her

are developing exercise programs in and out of the classroom to
expose kids to the benefits of exercise, without necessarily
making it seem like exercise. And one thing that they are
realizing is that an essential ingredient in any program is *you*.
In *The Family Fitness Handbook*, New York Road Runners
Club coach Bob Glover notes that the Swedes have a tradition of
regular family exercise days, on which parents and kids head off
for the mountains or the lake for a day of recreation. By comparison, our family gatherings these days seem to take place around
the TV set. So take a tip from the Swedes: Make exercise
something you do as a family, just like proper eating. Here are
some tips on how to do that, based on my own observations, plus
the experience of Vic Dante, who runs special fitness and stress-
management programs for kids.

Make it fun. Don't emphasize competition. Don't keep
score. Don't place emphasis on being faster or stronger or being
able to do more of something. Just try to have fun, whatever the
activity. "If you impose strict rules or goals, it becomes another
chore, another math test," says Dante. "Instead, try to make
your exercise time with your child a happy time, a fun time."

Lighten up, loosen up. Create a relaxed atmosphere for
family exercise. That starts with breathing. Encourage your
child to breathe slowly and deeply from the diaphragm, and to
move in a fluid, free-flowing way, whatever the activity.

Never force, strain, or push to the limit. How often do you see
Little League or Pee Wee football games and practices, in
which little boys are being badgered by their coaches to perform as if they're adults? I'm afraid I see it all too often. Let
me tell you, this "no pain, no gain" stuff is nonsense. These
days, even serious athletes know that they need to train, not
strain. They have to listen to their bodies. This applies to kids
especially. They shouldn't be pushed, by you or anybody else,
to the point of exhaustion. "Don't let your kids get into this

bust-a-gut macho mindset," says Dante. "They need to learn that you should feel good after a workout, not as if you've been run over by a truck."

Being active is more important than being involved in a specific activity. As adults, we have preconceived notions of what exercise is, whether it's running, racquetball, or a calisthenics regimen. That's not so with kids. Dancing to music videos can be a fun and fine exercise, even if it doesn't look like the kind of exercise you did in gym class. Conversely, notes Dante, "What looks good to you might seem nerdy to them. Kids are very style-conscious. Fine. Let them dance to their music. And their steps." The key is that whatever activity you (or they) choose, make sure it conforms to these general exercise rules:

• Aerobic exercise for kids—which is what we're talking about here—should be a brisk and sustained motion for at least twenty minutes three times a week—or better yet, thirty minutes four to five times a week. This will elevate their heart rate and burn calories without burning them out or putting undue stress on developing muscles.

• Make sure you precede each activity period with a five-minute warm-up of light, gradual stretching and finish up with a five-minute cool-down.

While the muscles are working, a metabolic process is going on, the end product of which is the formation of lactic acid. During normal activity, the circulation can keep up with the removal of this acid for disposal, but when the activity is greater, as during exercise, it piles up. A little time (during the "cool-down") is needed to complete the job. Left in the muscles, this lactic acid causes contractions (cramps). These are similar to those leg pains that some of our more active children complain about during the night.

• Wait on the weights. As I said before, using weights to get stronger is fine for adults and even teenagers, but not for

children. For them, exercising with weights should be avoided because it causes too much stress on the ends of their long bones, which are still growing, just as throwing curve balls can injure the young elbows of Little League pitchers. Postpone these activities until the growth plates in the bones are closed, which is when growth is completed. For those ten-year-olds who really want to look like Batman or Arnold, we think push-ups and sit-ups, both strength-building exercises that use their own body weight as resistance, are fine. But we would be surprised if they kept it up for long; there are much more fun ways to exercise for kids.

• Don't be perfect. This gets back to the philosophy behind our exercise program for your child. It's not about doing better, it's not about doing things "right," and no one is grading their performance. Dante recommends, and I agree, that we take the pressure off kids to do "well." They're doing well just by doing their exercise activities. Praise them for that, and join in.

Finally, what kid of exercise activities should you do? The sky's the limit, as Lesley showed me. In his book, Glover lists many creative possibilities, including games as familiar as hide-and-seek (emphasis on the *seek*, with all its running around), ring-o-levio, and activities as unstructured as gentle wrestling with your kids. You can contact your local YMCA or YMHA for ideas, too.

9

Infants, Toddlers, and Teens

Special Times, Special Considerations

Throughout most of the book, we've been focusing on children from the ages of two to about fourteen. Now let's turn our attention to what we might call the bookends of childhood: infancy, from birth to two, and the dreaded adolescent years, from thirteen to — in the case of some people I know — about thirty-five.

Seriously, both of these age groups, as well as the "toddler" stage, require special considerations when it comes to cholesterol, because babies and teens both undergo profound physiological changes. These changes directly affect how we deal with cholesterol at each of these ages.

INFANCY

Ask pediatricians about cholesterol and infants, and they'll say, "Don't even think about it for the first two years." As proof, they'll point to breast milk, which is very high in fat and cholesterol, and they'll tell you that's what Mother Nature intended.

Basically, I agree. I don't want to recommend any dietary restrictions for infants, but I think you should know that there is room for further study in this area. Just as a great deal of the medical "wisdom" about cholesterol and children has changed dramatically since the early 1970s, so may our views about cholesterol and infants change in the years to come.

I say this because we lack any solid evidence proving that infants actually *need* all that fat. Breast milk contains 40 to 45 percent fat—putting it on a par with McDonald's french fries. Why is it so high? Perhaps, some say, for the same reason that babies are still able to grasp with their feet as well as their hands. As you may have noticed, that's hardly a necessity in the modern world, but back in the days when our ancestors were still swinging from branches, a nimble foot was as important as a firm grip.

Some theorize that the high content of fat in breast milk is part of the same kind of prehistoric survival mechanism. Back then, the development of the central nervous system—the tissue that is formed by the fat in an infant's diet—may have been a greater concern than the risk of heart disease, which tends to come later in life—at an age you wouldn't reach if you didn't have reflexes fast enough to avoid being eaten by a saber-toothed tiger.

In another view, consuming high fat content *early* in life teaches the body how to deal with a high-fat diet *later* in life. In other words, according to this "cheeseburger theory," mother's milk is a way of preparing a child for all of the scrambled eggs, milkshakes, and cheeseburgers to come.

These, I should stress, are just theories. Although interesting, neither of them, in my mind, has conclusively answered the question of why breast milk has such a high fat content when excessive fat has been clearly shown to have adverse effects on humans as we get older. The bottom line is that infancy is a time of explosive growth, and dietary fat is important in that growth process. So, although breast milk does have a negative affect on cholesterol levels — it can even raise an infant's LDL — we still can't overlook its importance as an early nutrient.

For now, then, we must accept that breast milk is nature's way. But cheeseburgers aren't. So my advice is ultimately consistent with that of the rest of my colleagues. Let nature take its course for the first two years, and then let's work to keep pure and healthy what nature, and you, have created.

TODDLERS

Parents often come to me worried that their toddler is a "poor eater," and I tell them that they're right, but it's nothing to worry about. Most toddlers are notoriously miserable at the table — erratic, unpredictable, and even combative.

Why is this? Partially because of the dramatic slowing of the growth rate. They may seem to be shooting up like weeds to us, but growth is relative. The average three-year-old will grow only another 2 to 3 inches in the next year, compared to about 10 inches in the first year of life, and 4 inches during the second.

Another reason for the problem eating habits of toddlers is psychological, and seemingly paradoxical. Children of this age often try to manipulate their parents as a test of their own emerging sense of independence, and at the same time, they conform to the eating patterns around them. They seem more interested in playing than in eating, and yet they'll combine foods in seemingly bizarre — or, shall we say, creative — ways, such as having peanut butter and carrots for breakfast.

Keep in mind that these are normal patterns for children of this age group, and try not to get too frustrated. Instead, take a deep breath and remember:

1. The idea that we shouldn't snack between meals *doesn't* apply to toddlers. Indeed, snacks *are* their meals, as they have to eat more often to satisfy their fast-changing nutritional needs. Allow for regular snacking. Lightly cooked vegetables, peeled fruit slices, raw carrot sticks, and dry breakfast cereals are all healthy choices.

2. Always offer at least one food at a meal that the child likes, preferably one that is lower in fat.

3. Stay calm! If part or even all of the food is left untouched on your child's plate, its OK. Your child's body is a pretty efficient little mechanism. It knows, even better than you or I, just how much or how little fuel it needs to keep your toddler running at full speed.

4. Understand that it is normal for toddlers to have food jags for short stretches of time, so if your child seems to want to eat nothing but tuna fish and bananas for a week, be patient.

5. Be tolerant of slow eating. In fact, we should only hope that this is a habit your child will maintain past the toddler years.

6. Athletes have a saying: "Listen to your body." In the case of a toddler's eating habits, my recommendation is to listen to *their* bodies, and let them react accordingly. Toddlers will eat what they need, when they need it.

So relax, and enjoy these years. Finicky eating is natural for three-year-olds. Indeed, it's the least of the problems we should have as parents.

ADOLESCENCE

Now, let's fast-forward. If you're reading this part of the book, breast feeding, sleeping babies, even finicky-eating toddlers are probably a pleasant, distant memory. Now, you're dealing with a very different animal: the teenager. It's a difficult time in life, as we all know. Some of these difficulties will affect our goal: to help chart a lifetime course of good habits and a healthy heart. In most white male teenagers, the level of total cholesterol drops slightly before rising again in the late teens and early twenties. However, the reduction is in the "good" HDLs, while LDLs tend to rise. (Curiously, this is not the case in white females or in blacks, whose LDL levels drop during adolescence.)

What's more, some of the unhealthy practices that teenagers tend to experiment with—such as smoking, drinking, alcohol, and using oral contraceptives—have been shown to raise LDLs and lower HDLs even further. So preventive cholesterol treatments for teens should start with a reemphasis on the overall dangers of these other behaviors.

SMOKING

It's estimated that 30 to 40 percent of all teenagers smoke, but they're not as dumb as that statistic might indicate. Most teenagers these days know full well what the dangers of smoking are. They do it for other reasons, the chief one among them being peer approval.

There's a price to pay, of course, for looking "cool." Among all the other nasty things it does, adolescent smoking, even moderate smoking, has been shown to have a long-term effect on the development of atherosclerosis. It reduces the good

HDL and increases the bad VLDL (as you'll remember from Chapter 2, that's very-low-density lipoprotein). The effect is worse in girls than in boys, and even greater when the smoker also uses oral contraceptives.

How do you discourage smoking? By example, of course. If smoking stops, the effects are reversible, and I'm trusting that you and your spouse *don't* smoke. Beyond that, I think we can work on some of the ancillary motivations for smoking: stress and weight control. Lighting up isn't the only way to chill out or slim down. That's something you can teach your adolescent, and it may be an effort in which you find allies in your school district. Many schools now have antismoking programs involving peer group discussions using something every teenager can relate to: videos.

As far as peer pressure is concerned, it's tough. You can have only a limited role in that. However, I feel that the young people who play a more extensive role in this area — TV stars, rock musicians, and the like — need to be more aware of the effect they have on their impressionable audiences. Many, to their credit, are cognizant of these responsibilities, but many others continue to flaunt the habit. No, I'm not saying that you can get the lead guitarist of your son's favorite rock band or the lead heartthrob in the latest teenage soap opera to quit smoking, but I do know that a few angry letters to a network or record company can work wonders.

TELEVISION

Concern about television's messages leads us to the medium itself. A much-publicized study in 1991 by Dr. Kurt Gold at the University of California, Irvine, found that youngsters who watch more than two hours of TV a day are twice as likely to

have high cholesterol as those who don't. Sixty-five percent of
the excessive TV viewers were found to have cholesterol levels
over 170, and 53 percent had levels over 200. The box itself isn't
raising cholesterol, of course. It's what our children do—or
don't do—while they're sitting in front of that tube that's the
problem. Gold cited such things as unhealthy snacking while
viewing, exposure to frequent ads pushing high-fat junk foods,
and the obvious fact that excessive TV viewers are more sedentary. To make matters worse, a recent study found that metabolism slows while one is watching TV, so we burn those calories
even more slowly.

ORAL CONTRACEPTIVES

Like smoking, the use of oral contraceptives raises total
cholesterol and LDL levels while reducing HDL levels, and the
effects are synergistic. We don't know why, but the greater the
estrogen content of the pill, the worse the effect on cholesterol.
Interestingly, teenage girls' own estrogen has the opposite
effect, increasing HDL levels and decreasing VLDL levels. To
minimize the effect of oral contraceptives, eat healthy, don't
smoke, and use a low-estrogen pill.

OBESITY

An estimated 15 percent of teenagers are obese, and the
percentage is increasing. What are some of the reasons? Unhealthy eating habits, increased TV viewing, and inactivity are
three of the major ones. In addition to being associated with
high blood pressure, obesity can also lead to high LDL and
lower HDL levels.

ALCOHOL

The last thing you want your teenagers to believe is that drinking is somehow good for them. And yet, there is some evidence that the moderate consumption of alcohol may be linked to reduced heart-attack risk, by lowering cholesterol levels.

A now-famous study in this area was done in France. It concluded that the low heart-attack rates of the French could be attributed to their higher consumption of wine. This may sound like a convenient rationale to enjoy an extra glass of chablis or a beer. It shouldn't. The reporting of these kinds of studies in the mass media, eye-catching as they may be to the public, generally distorts or oversimplifies the findings. The French study, for example, raises a host of unanswered questions. For example, were the subjects on a generally low-fat diet for many years during and following World War II? Do the French — or at least the subjects in this particular study — consume fewer dairy products, fewer eggs, or less red meat? Are they less sedentary? On the other hand, do they have more automotive deaths, more cirrhosis of the liver, more pancreatic disorders, and an increased risk of cancer? We also know that heavy drinking increases cholesterol levels.

Teenagers need to learn responsible drinking habits. What they don't need is another excuse to drink excessively. Heavy alcohol consumption is not a solution to the cholesterol problem. It's simply another problem.

TEMPERAMENT

It has long been assumed that hard-driving, impatient, Type A personalities have a higher risk of suffering heart attacks, but new studies at Duke and Yale universities cast

doubt on this theory. They find that the more dangerous type
of personality in terms of heart disease is a hostile and angry
person.

This startling finding was determined by observing the
reactions of college students when they were continually, and
deliberately, bothered by a tester while trying to solve word
puzzles. The more hostile subjects reacted with anger and
higher blood pressure. When measured, these students were
found to have higher cholesterol and lower HDL levels. On
further examination, it was found that they also tended to have
other unhealthy lifestyles, like smoking and poor eating habits.
When followed up in later years, the more hostile subjects were
three times likelier to develop heart disease, and five times
more at risk if they also had high cholesterol levels. Dr. Redford
Williams of Duke commented, "People with high hostility at
age 19 tend to have high cholesterol at 40."

What are the implications of this research? Although we
can't begin to examine here all the causes leading to anger or
hostility in a teenager, we can at least be aware of the possible
connection between that kind of personality and health problems, and *that's* the first step in dealing with these problems.

Clearly, adolescents seem drawn to the kinds of habits and
behaviors associated with higher cholesterol levels and heart
disease in later life. This is particularly important because it's
during the teenage years that long-term lifestyle habits — such
as diet, smoking, and drinking — are established.

So what can you do to try to steer your teenager toward
healthier habits? Here are some of my thoughts:

• Teenagers, it seems, are always hungry. And with good
reason. They have a sudden and explosive need for more
calories and energy during these maturing years. "Got anything
to eat?" is their constant refrain. And your response, at least at
home, should be to have healthy foods readily available.

• Try to involve your teenager in menu planning, food
shopping, and food preparation. Besides being a good preparation for life — and all teenagers claim to be waiting for that great
day when they can live on their own — it's a way to begin helping
them recognize their responsibility for what goes into their own
bodies. Furthermore, it would provide an all-too-rare time for
you and your teen to talk about something other than grades,
college, and whether or not she or he can have the car. In this
case, the topic would be nutrition.

• Latchkey kids — those who come home to an empty
house after school — need special attention. We know that children who eat alone tend to eat a more unhealthy diet. For these
youngsters, then, it's especially important to have the fresh
fruits and vegetables, bagels, and whole grains available — the
grab-and-go foods that they can eat "unsupervised."

• My best advice in dealing with teenagers and their
health is to take advantage of their susceptibility to peer pressure, and of their interest in and concern with their bodies and
their looks. Healthy eating, exercise, and other aspects of a
healthy lifestyle can be emphasized as a way to feel and look
good — particularly to the opposite sex (something teenagers
are becoming all too aware of). In the end, no young person
I've ever known really *wanted* to be fat.

10

What We Can Learn from a Pediatric Cholesterol Center

The program described in this book is the one I recommend to all of my patients and their families. But in some cases, I feel that closer supervision may be necessary.

When a child's total cholesterol level is measured at over 200, the first thing I do is put him or her on a low-fat diet for three months and then retest. If the levels are still over 200, I refer the parents to the hyperlipidemia center at Schneider Children's Hospital of Long Island Jewish Hospital, a major local hospital.

I think we can all learn from the way the people at Schneider and other pediatric centers around the country deal with their patients. I'm not saying you need to send your child to such a clinic. You probably don't. But if your pediatrician recommends it, don't panic. These are not cardiac care wards, where your child will be treated like a heart patient. *Hyperlipidemia* simply means elevated levels of fat; it doesn't mean anyone is about to have a heart attack.

Indeed, what they preach at these clinics is very similar to what you've read in this book. The only difference is that, for the four hundred or so children referred to Schneider, the odds are greater of developing heart disease in later life if—big *if*—they don't begin making diet and lifestyle modifications.

Generally, the procedures followed at Schneider are similar to those at most clinics. The director of the center, Dr. Marc Jacobson, was gracious enough to invite me in to spend a morning with Nancy Copperman, a registered dietician at the center.

When I arrived, I was amazed by how pleasant it was. The atmosphere was nonthreatening. Everybody was warm and pleasant. I felt reassured and secure in the knowledge that the many patients I'd referred here over the years were being well taken care of.

Ms. Copperman is typical of the kind of professional you'll find at a center like this. She was up to date on the latest research, well informed, and able to get crucial information across to parents in an understandable way. I found her to be a no-nonsense, battle-tested pro, and her experiences and thoughts on the war against cholesterol were so useful that I wanted to share our conversation with you:

Q: Nancy, centers like yours pride themselves on a team approach. Can you tell us about the members of your team?

A: We have our director, Dr. Jacobson, who is also a pediatrician and sees patients. He has an associate physician who also works with us. We have two dieticians, including myself, a lab technician, and a behavioral psychologist who specializes in child development and works with some of our patients.

Q: Your evaluation starts before the child even sets foot in the clinic. Correct?

A: Yes. We have a family history form for our patients to fill out, which goes through both sides of the family, mother's and father's. This includes aunts, uncles, grandparents, siblings, all the way down the line. We ask questions about strokes, about angina, about heart attacks, myocardial infarctions, and hypertension. We ask them to indicate the age at which these events occurred, as best they know. The physician reviews this information and, when the parents come in, goes over it again with them to help fill in the blanks.

Q: What about diet? Do they fill out a form for that as well?

A: Yes. We ask them to fill out a three-day diet diary— everything the child has eaten or drunk for three days.

Q: So all of this is done *before* the parents actually come into the center. What happens then?

A: After a routine physical examination and a check of the child's growth records, the first thing we do is reassure the parents that their child is healthy. He or she is not here because we're afraid he or she is going to have a heart attack tomorrow, but because we all want to prevent something that might happen in the future. I'm amazed at how many parents don't understand that. They really think that their child is about to have a heart attack.

Q: So, that's the first step. Reassurance.

A: Right. And we remind our patients that no matter what their family history looks like, these kids are much better off because, if there is any predisposition that seems to be in the family, it's been discovered.

Q: I'm often surprised at how many parents don't know their *own* cholesterol levels. Do you find that also?

A: If they don't know, we encourage them very strongly to find out. Because if there *is* a problem, it's a more urgent issue for them. After all, the parents may have been walking around with high cholesterol levels for decades, as opposed to how long their children have. In fact, we had one case where a father didn't know his cholesterol levels, and we told him that he should get them checked. He did, and two weeks later he was in the hospital for a triple bypass. He came back and said, "You saved my life."

Q: Family involvement in a healthy diet really starts at home, doesn't it?

A: Absolutely. Dad can't bring Haagen Dazs home while the kid's eating Sealtest Free. If the parents are eating right, you'll have better compliance by the child.

Q: The reason we're doing this book is to educate parents. Do you find that you're doing a lot of educating here?

A: Yes, and one way we do it is with our monthly "Family Night," when we invite all of the family members: grandparents, aunts, uncles, friends, and the kids. We give them an hour-long presentation, explaining our dietary goals and our approach to diet, explaining about cholesterol and fats. It's an effort to give them some basic education and make them understand how important they are in this process.

Q: What is your approach to diet?

A: We give parents some basic guidelines. We tell them they need to limit their meat, chicken, fish, and cheese to about 5 to 7 ounces a day, explaining that a portion is about the size of a deck of cards. If you're going to go for second portions, go for the carbohydrates and not a second helping of meat. Most people can grasp that.

Q: Do you use the substitution method?

A: Yes, and I'll give you some specific examples. Instead of beef franks, we tell parents to use turkey franks. We say instead of one cookie you can have, say, seventeen "Teddy Grahams" (little Graham crackers). Then we give them a list of what we call "free foods," foods that have no fat or cholesterol in them at all, like pretzels, air-popped popcorn, fruits, fruit rollups, bread, and bagels. There are no limits on these foods.

Q: You talk about "visible" and "invisible" foods. Can you explain that?

A: Take eggs, for example. Visible eggs are used in home and outside food preparations — scrambled eggs, eggs over easy, or things that you dip a cutlet in. We tell parents to take the yolks out of these visible eggs but use all of the whites they want. Once they do that, they don't have to worry about scanning labels for the "invisible" eggs, because who can figure out how much of an egg yolk is in a cookie, anyway?

Q: How do you advise them when it comes to reading labels?

A: We tell them that, when they see something that says "cholesterol free" on a food, just ignore it, because, until all of the new labeling guidelines are fully in effect, it means little. We tell them that cholesterol can come only from an animal and therefore is found only in animal products.

Q: Are there foods that you strictly prohibit?

A: We've found that if you make foods forbidden, then the children tend to want them even more. So Mom might send them to school with a turkey sandwich, and they trade it for bologna anyway.

Q: What do you feel about oat bran's place in the diet, and how do you counsel parents about it?

A: First of all, none of the studies that showed the purported value of oat bran were done on children, and a study that came out of Columbia University more recently showed that the cholesterol-lowering effect was due mainly to the displacement of fat *per se*; that is, the people who happened to be eating oat bran were also eating less fat in their diet and *that* was why their cholesterol was lowered. It was not necessarily because of the oat bran. Now, that's not to say oat bran isn't good. We tell parents it's a good adjunct and a good source of fiber, but we advise them not just to go buying things with oat bran in them, as if it were some kind of magic cure, because it certainly isn't. And it can almost be counterproductive, especially when you see all these so-called oat bran cakes, potato chips, and muffins that may have 20 grams of fat in them and just a trace of oat bran.

Q: Speaking of miracle cures, what about fish oils? They got a lot of attention for a while, too.

A: We're very much against fish oils for children for several reasons. First, when you call the companies that manufacture these supplements and ask them where the fish that provide the oils are coming from, no one can or will tell you. So, if they came from toxic waters, these poisons are going to be dissolved in the fish oils, which you're going to be giving to children. Also, too much fish oil can result in impaired clotting and prolonged bleeding. Third, you run a risk of overdosing on fat-soluble vitamins. So, if you're giving your child lots of cod liver oil, as some parents do, you could have a problem. Finally, we have to remember that fish oils themselves are pure fat, and the thrust of our entire program is to reduce fat in the diet.

Q: As part of your approach to lowering cholesterol among children, do you encourage fitness, exercise, and weight control?

A: If the child is obese, part of the plan is to get her or him involved in aerobic exercise, though not necessarily in a structured program. We encourage kids to run, bike, swim, and even play hockey. Some of our kids just walk around the block or up and down the stairs of their apartment building. Basically, we just encourage them to start moving!

Q: Let's get on to a ticklish subject: drugs. Parents aren't very receptive to the idea. We're not quick to use them. What do you do here at the center?

A: We *do* use drugs to lower cholesterol, in exceptional cases. These are the criteria: first, if there are inadequate results from diet alone, after six months to a year under our super-vision; second, if there is a very strong family history, that is, where one parent has had symptoms of heart disease or has actually died; and third, if their LDL level is above the 95th percentile. Then and only then will we consider a child a candidate for such cholesterol-lowering drugs as choles-tyramine and colestipol, which have few side effects.

Q: And what are your results with the drugs?

A: The results are good. Out of the four hundred or so patients we see here, maybe only five or six are on drug therapy. What we see on average is a reduction of 10 to 15 percent in total cholesterol. And remember that 10 to 15 percent for a kid with a total cholesterol level of over 300 is a significant drop. They remain on the drugs as long as necessary, until changes in diet and lifestyle can take over.

Q: Do any children ever come to surgery for this problem?

A: Now *that's* one in a million. The kids who might be candi-dates for surgery have "homozygous familial hypercholes-terolemia." These are kids whose cholesterol levels may be up in the thousands. They're really sick, and in the past, most didn't survive past age twelve. Now we have proce-dures, such as lipodialysis, that clean the blood of its excess fat. It's similar to the way waste products are removed from the blood in kidney dialysis, and it's improving the odds for many of these children.

Q: In a recent journal paper, a prominent endocrinologist ex-pressed concern about the possibility of growth being stunted by diet restrictions. I know you're aware of his study. What are your reactions to it?

A: First, he used only a few children in this study, an ex-tremely small sample on which to be making judgments. We followed 100 patients on low-fat–low-cholesterol diets for three years and found normal growth in weight and height as well as measures of fat and muscle among these children, compared with other children of a similar age. Therefore, we have every reason to believe that low-fat–low-cholesterol diets can support normal growth in children.

Q: It's a tough thing to generalize, I know, but what kind of results are you getting?

A: As you point out, kids are going to respond in different ways, but a 15 to 20 percent reduction in total cholesterol is what you expect from diet modification, and that's what we're getting, usually in less than a year.

Q: Fifteen to twenty percent reduction? That's very good. It's almost twice as high as I would have expected. It suggests to me that we have a lot to learn, and a lot to unlearn. You've heard a lot of myths about kids and cholesterol, haven't you?

A: I sure have. Myth 1: Veal is better for you than beef, even though it comes from the same animal. Myth 2: Animal fats are more hazardous to your health than vegetable fats. The truth is that you're better off eating lard than coconut or palm oil! Myth 3: We'll go on the diet for six months and the problem will be solved, and then we can go back to our greasy hamburgers and french fries again.

Q: Of course, it's a lifetime commitment, but that raises an important question: How often do you see your patients?

A: It depends on the age, and it depends on how high the cholesterol level is. Generally, we see them once every three months to begin with, and depending on how well they're doing, we can gradually stretch the interval up to annual visits that may continue through adolescence.

Q: Speaking of myths, I'll add one more myself: Clinics like yours are last resorts, that they're somber, and that the kids here are guinea pigs or children destined for a lifetime of heart problems. That's all nonsense, and the proof is in the results you cited to me, and in the feedback I get from parents I've referred to you. Thanks for your time.

11

Getting Your Kids to Say "Yes"

I never lie to my young patients, but sometimes, I must confess, I have to distract them. When I'm about to have a young child shot, I step gently on his foot. When he looks down, whammo. He gets his shot and a "hero" sticker slapped on his shirt for the good behavior he didn't even have time to realize that he demonstrated.

I think the same principle can be applied to the diet and lifestyle changes you've learned about in this book. The technical word is *compliance*. What that really means is getting your kids to say the magic word: *yes*.

So how do we do it? Well, there are a number of suggestions I can give, starting with my "distraction" method. Just as we crafty pediatricians will draw a child's attention away from the big, bad needle—for their own good, of course—I think you might similarly "distract" your child from the notion that the foods you're preparing for them are "healthy" foods. The word *healthy* makes it sound suspiciously like medicine, which is something no child wants any part of.

Try putting things in their terms, instead. I do. In fact, I

167

talk to the children about the importance of a low-fat diet, and they respond, as long as it's been put in a positive, nonthreatening way. So, rather than telling them that the low-fat diet will keep their cholesterol level down or that it's good for their hearts or that it will keep them from getting sick someday—concepts that are difficult and even frightening to an eight-year-old—talk to them in an upbeat way and in terms they can understand.

Kids are very competitive. Eating this kind of food, you might tell them, will help them run faster and grow bigger and stronger. They'll look better. They'll feel better. They'll do better in games, in sports, and in school.

There is no shortage of available role models to help illustrate your point. When I was a kid, it was Popeye and his spinach, or whoever was on the Wheaties box that month. Today, it could be Joe Montana or Michael Jordan, if your kids are into sports. Or, as I ask some of my little ones, do you really think Batman could be big and strong and fast enough to catch the Joker and all of his allies if he didn't eat the right food? And, of course (although I haven't really been able to look into Batman's refrigerator to see if he's following the Step One diet), all of this is *true*. Eating these good, tasty foods *will* make them feel better and do better. Now, here are some other tips:

Never say never. If your children do what you want them to do (in this case, eat the foods you want them to eat), give them praise. If they don't, let it pass. Remember what we've said all along in this book. Occasional junk food is OK; a junk food diet is not. You *can* have a birthday cake for your child's birthday as long as you compensate for it. As Dr. James Cleeman, coordinator of the National Cholesterol Education Program, says, "It's not about never eating certain foods or that certain foods are bad. It's a matter of making the entire eating pattern a sound one."

Try to stay a step ahead of them. The most effective way to get your children to eat right is to limit the number of opportunities for them to eat incorrectly. If you've filled your kitchen with good, wholesome, low-fat foods, they have no choice but to make a good choice. When they come in hungry, you should have something ready—something that they'll eat because they *are* hungry. And maybe, by eating it, they'll see that Mommy and Daddy were right, and it *does* taste good.

Make it fun to eat right. Even adults tend to think that eating foods that are good for you means eating foods that are dull and tasteless. As I hope you've found in the past few chapters, nothing could be further from the truth (and if you need some more proof, see the sample recipes at the end of this book).

Show your kids that this isn't just good food; it's also food that tastes great. Use colorful foods, and what could be more colorful than a rainbow of so-called boring vegetables or multicolored pastas? Make the food look fun, even festive. Use small portions on large plates, especially if the food is unfamiliar.

Use the familiarity principle. Familiarity is an important word. Children like familiar things—and are suspicious of strange and new things. I learned this lesson myself the day that my four-year-old son walked into our kitchen as dinner was being prepared, sniffed the air, and announced, "Whatever it is I smell, I'm not eating it."

How do you get around this problem? Start young, and start small. If it's too late to start your child young, it's never too late to start making the gradual changes that add up to a healthy diet.

A new diet—one that your child will accept—isn't built overnight. Take your time. Make small, incremental changes. Introduce new foods within the context of foods that your child is already comfortable with. You can go from serving, say, a plateful of corn and a speck of broccoli to a dish that's half corn and half broccoli. But take your time. If one pushes, I've found, children will recoil.

On the other side of the coin, delete fatty foods from the diet at the same deliberate pace. Don't suddenly announce, "No more ice cream!" Gradually cut back, from two scoops to one, or from three ice cream desserts a week to one. From there, you can move to ice milk or low-fat frozen yogurt. Use the substitution table in Chapter 4 (pp. 82–84) for suggestions, and remember that you can't force a good diet on anyone, especially your child.

Don't give guilt; give good-tasting food. Parents say to me all the time, "My child just won't eat for me." I reply to this Freudian slip, "That's because they're not eating to please *you*. They're eating for themselves." Don't use guilt as a way to get your child to eat the way you want him or her to. Simply offer good food that tastes good. The rest is up to the child.

For a responsible, concerned parent like yourself, I know that's easier said than done. But remember, you can only do so much. You're learning about the right foods. You're going to start buying and preparing the right foods. You're offering the right foods. You're being a good parent by doing all of that. But that's all you *can* do.

Make mealtime a peaceful time. I know it may sound old-fashioned, but to me, mealtime is a time to eat meals. It's not a time to watch TV, scold your child, or argue.

Mealtime, I think, should have a positive aura. It shouldn't be a time when kids worry that Mom will yell at them about homework. The child who sits down at the table every night with a knotted stomach is going to have trouble eating anything, including the good foods we want her or him to eat. Save the harangues for times other than mealtime.

We don't encourage combining TV viewing with eating. Many studies have shown that kids who watch a great deal of TV are often overweight and have higher cholesterol levels.

So turn off the TV, and don't bring up the unpleasantries. Make mealtimes a pleasant, relaxed time — the ideal environment for serving and discovering new foods and for encouraging good eating habits.

Get your child involved in the diet. School-aged kids want to start doing things themselves. They're becoming more independent, and they want to be able to do the things you do. So let them. Involve them in food planning and preparation. You can make a game of it. Take them to the supermarket, and ask them to find all of the foods that are low-fat, or at least that say so on the label. Then ask them to find a food that labels itself "high-fat." Of course, they'll look high and low without finding a single such item. Now they've learned not only how smart you are, but that the food companies know how smart you are. They've also learned a lesson about selling, as opposed to truth.

Get them involved in the cooking as well. Let them experiment with new seasonings, new preparations, and new ingredients. This is not only an excellent way to "field-test" substitutions, but it's also a great way to get compliance. Because chances are, if they feel that they helped make the meal, they're going to be more likely to eat and enjoy it.

The whole point here is that you're trying to let your children feel that they have some control, which is, after all, as essential lesson of growing up.

When all else fails, and your child comes to you screaming for Teenage Mutant Ninja Turtle cereal, or some other sugar-laden concoction she or he has seen on TV or been served at a friend's house, how do you deal with it? Talk about it. Don't say no. Say, "OK, but . . ." Let your children know that they can have this cereal, *but* it's not the best one and they should agree to try those that are better. Then follow that plan. Let them have their sugar cereal, but gradually "dilute" it with a healthier choice, increasing its percentage until what they're eating has gone from bad to good.

And what if you catch them jumping up and down in front of the TV over a commercial for a candy bar? Do you switch off the TV or change the channel to educational programming? No. Let them watch it, and then talk to them about it. Kids don't understand that TV commercials and, unfortunately, many TV programs for kids are not aimed at informing or even entertaining them. Their goal is purely and simply to sell a product.

Kids should be told that advertisements — like labels — are not necessarily the unvarnished truth. Explain that the products being advertised are not necessarily good for them. This explanation may not click in at first, but with repetition, it will. Your child will begin to understand the distinction — and may begin to watch commercials in the same skeptical way we all should.

You handle a food tantrum the same way you handle any other kind of tantrum. First, let it pass. Don't intervene. When it's over, understanding begins — in a calmer atmosphere. At first, you may not realize how successful you have been, but after repetition and reinforcement, learning will occur. We reminded you a moment ago about how little control parents have over their children's appetite, their metabolism, and their physiology. Where parents exert an enormous amount of control, however (and therefore, I think, have an important responsibility), is on their child's psychology: what they perceive, what they learn, what they think, and ultimately what they come to believe.

As any teacher or coach will tell you, the essence of learning is simplification and repetition. If your children understand that eating a certain way will make them feel, look, and perform better, and if that message is repeated, not once or twice, but over the course of months and years, they'll ultimately get it. And you may someday have the satisfaction of hearing your child repeat the same advice to his or her little friend — or your own grandchild.

DIETING FOR THE OBESE CHILD

We conclude with the topic of the obese child because submitting to a diet is a form of compliance. However, when it comes to weight loss diets for children, I can sum up my recommendations in one word: Don't.

Most of the experts feel that weight loss diets — and weight loss summer camps, I should add — are counterproductive for children. Why? Because all too often these diets are forced on children. True weight loss occurs only when the motivation comes from within the child, and when the desire is brought on by peer pressure, social goals, athletic goals, and the goal of pure self-satisfaction. That is the best way to avoid the "bounce" syndrome: the cycle of fat to thin to even-fatter-than-ever that we see so often in unmotivated obese children.

The key to working with obese children is not to let them go hungry — or *think* they're going hungry. You select the foods. You select the mealtimes. Let the child decide how *much* to eat. Even the child who continues to gorge for a while will eventually learn to trust the diet, to lose the fear that many psychologists feel is one basis of obesity in children: the fear of not getting enough to eat.

In general, I think obese children benefit greatly from a low-cholesterol diet, and not only because obesity and cholesterol levels are often (but not always) related. Remember that fat has more than twice the calories of carbohydrates and protein, so by following a low-fat diet, no only will we be lowering these children's cholesterol, but we'll also automatically be reducing their caloric intake.

12

Keeping Up with Changes

Recently, a special-education teacher I know gave a long and serious lecture on nutrition. At the conclusion of her talk, she asked the class what they had learned. A boy in the back waved his hand furiously and, when recognized, said, "I learned that if the salt don't getcha, the sugar will."

I know just what he meant. We pediatricians are bombarded with information disseminated by various food industry groups, universities, medical organizations, and pharmaceutical companies. I'm often left feeling that if the lovastatin doesn't get you, the cholestyramine will.

As you read this, researchers in universities, hospitals, foundations, and laboratories around the world are studying the issues we've been talking about in this book. And given the vital health issues at stake — not to mention the public interest in health, fitness, nutrition, and, of course, parenting — you can be sure a lot of the results will make their way into your daily newspaper or onto your local news program — and also into my mailbox.

How should you interpret these news reports, especially if they contradict some of the things you've read here or that your doctor has told you? First, take a page out of the medical practitioner's book. We have to pick and choose from a flood of material that comes across our desks. What makes sense, and what doesn't? What is useful, and what isn't? Our work depends on keeping abreast of the advances in the field. But to be honest, if we tried to change the way we practiced medicine based on every new report or every new study that's done, we'd have no time to practice. We'd be running around in circles, second-guessing ourselves.

That's why most doctors tend to lie back and wait for replication of the results by other researchers studying the same problem, and for confirmation that the new miracle cure or breakthrough discovery is really that—and not just a statistical quirk, a mistake in methodology, or an incorrect interpretation of the data.

Granted, there are some physicians who are *too* conservative. I'm not arguing for pigheadedness, just prudence. Although most doctors *are* hungry for information about new treatments that can make us more effective in our work, we know that for every ten claims made, only one will survive the test of time.

Why is the batting average so low? Partly because the mysteries of the human body yield solutions only gradually, but there's a more prosaic reason that has to do with the way research is conducted and who's paying for it. The first thing you might do when you read anything about a new medical development is to consider the source. You don't need me to tell you that there are great corporations in this country whose fortunes are tied to America's eating habits. For many of these companies, producers of the kinds of foods that have a high fat and cholesterol content, the new understanding of the relationship of these nutrients to heart disease—and the trend toward smarter, healthier diets—is a direct threat to business. They've counter-

attacked with their own research; research which may be conducted by a so-called independent scientist, but which is
usually done with the aim of finding results that are favorable
to the client. The name of the sponsor of such research is not
generally a company name, but the name of some trade association, council, or "institute." Make no mistake about it, these
are lobbying groups that exist solely to promote the use of these
products. So, if you read that a new study sponsored by the Beef
Council has found that eating red meat actually lowers cholesterol levels, take it with a grain of sodium chloride.

That's not to say that all research sponsored by something
with a commercial stake in the outcome is invalid. A recent
study funded by Quaker Oats, for example, found that oat bran
has no special cholesterol-lowering effect. This is certainly
not the result Quaker hoped for. On the other hand, research
done by sources in academia or independent organizations may
not be unslanted, either. "The peddler of a biased point of view
is as likely to be an anti-establishment crusader or an academic
ladder-climber as a corporate darling," noted *Washington Post*
science writer Vincent Cook in an *In Health* magazine story.

So whom do you believe? Of course, there is a great deal of
important work being done by respected and genuinely independent researchers, many of whom have made the discoveries
that the advice in this book is based on. How do you know what
to pay attention to? When should new research prompt you to
make changes in your diet or behavior? The answer is "rarely."
I agree with Jane Brody, the well-known author and health
writer for the *New York Times*, who said, "Don't let one study
change your life."

But in order to make your and your child's life a little
healthier and happier—and to keep you from wondering
whether it's the salt or the sugar that "gotcha"—here are some

questions you may want to ask yourself the next time some well-
meaning friend hands you a newspaper clipping about the latest
"ground-breaking" study on cholesterol:

Where does the story come from? Is it from a self-interest group
or a careful, serious source such as the Framingham Heart
Study, the Louisiana State University Bogalusa group, the
Centers for Disease Control (CDC), the National Cholesterol
Education Group, a major university, or major medical journal
such as the *Journal of the American Medical Association* (JAMA)?
If so, it should be given more weight.

These places have lofty reputations, which, in my opinion,
are well earned. Whether it's the CDC or the JAMA, these
organizations are dedicated to the painstaking process of scientific research. And the people who run them, whether they are
the directors of a major university teaching hospital who super-
vise the studies done in their labs or the board of experts who
review each of the articles submitted to the journals, are thoroughly grounded in the fundamentals of good research method-
ologies. These sources are stringent in upholding the standards
that guide our search for scientific truth.

*Was the sample used large enough to allow the drawing of
generalizations?* Not long ago, a representative of one of the
largest drug companies in the country came into my office,
claiming that an antibiotic his company makes works as well
given twice a day as it does given three times, an obvious
convenience. When I expressed skepticism, he mailed two
scientific studies to me "proving" this claim. Unfortunately,
they were based on only fifty-five and ninety patients, respec-
tively, with throat and ear infections — absurdly small samples
for such common illnesses. Worse yet, the studies found that the
cure rate was 81 percent — 7 percent higher than the average
cure rate with the *same* antibiotics given *three* times a day, an
impossibility that can be attributed only to the small sample size.

As my old statistics professor in college used to remind us, *percent* means for each 100, so I would recommend paying greater attention to long-term, large-sample studies. Although there is no absolute minimum required sample size for a valid study, my recommendation is that unless we're dealing with a sample size of a hundred subjects or more, we can reserve judgment.

Is it logical? You don't need a science degree to apply common sense. Is it likely that we can get hens to lay low-cholesterol eggs? That was a newspaper story out of Alberta, Canada, in 1990. But until those farmers show me an egg with less than 270 milligrams of cholesterol in its yolk, I'll stick to the whites, thank you.

Are they confusing cause with association? A researcher once reported a correlation between a drop in the price of corn with an increase in the number and severity of hayfever cases. Were all these people sneezing and sniffling because the price of corn went down? No. It was because corn is cheaper when there's a larger crop of corn, and the same weather conditions that are good for growing corn are also good for producing a bumper crop of ragweed!

Is this the last word on the subject—or the first? Jane Brody told *In Health* that she generally waits for three types of studies before changing her own eating habits. First, she looks for studies of large groups that demonstrate a link between a particular food and a particular health "effect." Then, she watches for lab evidence in test animals that suggests how the food causes its effect. Finally, she considers "blind" experiments, in which two groups of humans are compared, one eating the food and the other—a control group—not eating it, with *neither group knowing which is which.*

That's good advice. It reminds us that we shouldn't change our habits—or our children's—on the basis of one study. Wait to see if the findings are repeated in another study. If they are, and if the results are important enough, you'll hear about it. Then you can make an intelligent judgment.

Also, to help gauge the credibility of any given study reported in the mass media, look for quotes from other authorities outside the ones who conducted the experiment. A good journalist will seek the perspectives of well-known experts in the field — people who may not have been involved in the study, but who are familiar enough with all of the studies in this area to assess this study's significance.

In other words, don't buy the first story, don't embrace the first new "miracle" food, and don't rush to have your pediatrician prescribe the first new medication, whether it has to do with lowering your child's cholesterol level or curing the common cold. Do as we doctors do. Stand back. Think, watch, and wait. In the meantime, stick with the tried and true, which, I believe, is how we can characterize much of the information in this book. The advice, the diets, the techniques, and even the individual food substitutions have been tried by my colleagues, by my patients, and by me. We've found them to be sound — and hope you will, too. Good luck!

Food Tables

These alphabetically arranged food tables can be a useful tool when you are making food choices. They list calories, grams of fat, and grams of saturated fat as well as what percentage of the calories come from the fat and the saturated fat.

These tables are not definitive. Always read labels. When a label does not give the percentage of the calories that come from fat, you can figure it out with this simple equation:

grams of fat × 9 ÷ by the total number of calories per serving

There is also a list of high-fiber food. Research has shown that a diet high in fiber has a beneficial effect on cholesterol levels.

Item and serving	Calories	Total fat (grams)	% total fat	Saturated fat (grams)	% saturated fat	Cholesterol (milligrams)
FRUITS						
Apple						
w/peel, 1 medium	81	0.4	trace	0.1	trace	0
dried, ½ cup	155	0.1	tr.	0	0	0

181

Item and serving	Calo-ries	Total fat (grams)	% total fat	Satu-rated fat (grams)	% satu-rated fat	Choles-terol (milli-grams)
FRUITS (*cont.*)						
Applesauce, unsweetened, ½ cup	53	0.1	tr.	0	0	0
Apricots						
fresh, 3 medium	51	0.4	tr.	0	0	0
dried, 5 halves	83	0.3	tr.	0	0	0
Avocados						
California, 1 (6 oz.)	306	30.0	88	4.5	13	0
Florida, 1 (11 oz.)	339	27.0	71	5.3	14	0
Banana, 1 medium	105	0.6	tr.	0.2	tr.	0
Blackberries						
fresh, 1 cup	74	0.5	tr.	0	0	0
frozen, 1 cup	97	0.7	tr.	0	0	0
Blueberries						
fresh, 1 cup	82	0.6	tr.	0	0	0
frozen, 1 cup	80	0.7	tr.	0.2	tr.	0
Boysenberries						
canned, ½ cup	113	0.2	tr.	0	0	0
frozen, 1 cup	66	0.7	tr.	0	0	0
Breadfruit, ¼ small	99	0.2	tr.	0	0	0
Cantaloupe, 1 cup	57	0.4	tr.	0	0	0
Cherries						
maraschino, ¼ cup	56	0.1	tr.	0	0	0
sour, canned in heavy syrup, ½ cup	116	0.4	tr.	0	0	0
sweet, ½ cup	49	0.7	tr.	0.1	tr.	0
Cranberries, fresh, 1 cup	46	0.2	tr.	0	0	0

Item and serving	Calo-ries	Total fat (grams)	% total fat	Satu-rated fat (grams)	% satu-rated fat	Choles-terol (milli-grams)
FRUITS (cont.)						
Cranberry-orange relish, ½ cup	246	0.9	tr.	0	0	0
Cranberry sauce, ½ cup	209	0.2	tr.	0	0	0
Dates, whole, ½ cup	228	0.4	tr.	0	0	0
Figs						
fresh, 1 medium	37	0.2	tr.	0	tr.	0
dried, 10 figs	477	1.0	2	0.4	tr.	0
Fruit cocktail, 1 cup, canned in juice	112	0.3	tr.	0	0	0
Fruit leather, 1 piece	50	0	0	0	0	0
Grapefruit, ½ me-dium	39	0.1	tr.	0	0	0
Grapes, 10						
Thompson seed-less	35	0.3	tr.	0	0	0
red flame	40	0.2	tr.	0	0	0
Guava, 1 medium	45	0.3	tr.	0.2	tr.	0
Honeydew melon, ½ small	33	0.3	tr.	0	0	0
Kiwi, 1 medium	46	0.3	tr.	0	0	0
Kumquat, 1 me-dium	12	0	0	0	0	0
Lemon, 1 medium	17	0.2	tr.	0	0	0
Lime, 1 medium	20	0.1	tr.	0	0	0
Mandarin oranges, canned in juice, ½ cup	46	0.1	tr.	0	0	0
Mango, 1 medium	135	0.6	tr.	0.1	tr.	0

Item and serving	Calo-ries	Total fat (grams)	% total fat	Satu-rated fat (grams)	% satu-rated fat	Choles-terol (milli-grams)
FRUITS *(cont.)*						
Melon balls, 1 cup	55	0.4	tr.	0	0	0
Mixed fruit, dried, 1 cup	243	0.5	tr.	0	0	0
Mixed fruit, frozen and sweetened, 1 cup	245	0.5	tr.	0.2	tr.	0
Mulberries, fresh, 1 cup	61	0.6	tr.	0	0	0
Nectarine, 1 me-dium	67	0.6	tr.	0	0	0
Orange						
navel, 1 medium	65	0.2	tr.	0	0	0
Valencia, 1 me-dium	59	0.4	tr.	0	0	0
Papaya, 1 medium	117	0.4	tr.	0.1	tr.	0
Peach						
fresh, 1 medium	58	0.1	tr.	0	0	0
canned in heavy syrup, 1 cup	190	0.3	tr.	0	0	0
canned in light syrup, 1 cup	136	0.2	tr.	0	0	0
canned, water-packed, 1 cup	58	0.1	tr.	0	0	0
frozen, sweet-ened, 1 cup	235	0.3	tr.	0	0	0
Pear						
fresh, 1 medium	98	0.7	tr.	0	0	0
canned in heavy syrup, 1 cup	188	0.3	tr.	0	0	0
canned in light syrup, 1 cup	144	0.1	tr.	0	0	0

Item and serving	Calo-ries	Total fat (grams)	% total fat	Satu-rated fat (grams)	% satu-rated fat	Choles-terol (milli-grams)
FRUITS (cont.)						
Persimmon, 1 medium	32	0.1	tr.	0	0	0
Pineapple pieces, fresh, 1 cup	77	0.7	tr.	0	0	0
canned, unsweet-ened, 1 cup	150	0.2	tr.	0	0	0
Plum, 1 medium	36	0.6	tr.	0	0	0
canned in heavy syrup, 1 cup	104	0.5	tr.	0	0	0
Prunes, 10 whole	115	0.2	tr.	0	0	0
Raisins, ¼ cup						
dark seedless	112	0.1	tr.	0.1	tr.	0
golden	113	0.1	tr.	0.1	tr.	0
Raspberries						
fresh, 1 cup	61	0.2	tr.	0	0	0
frozen, sweet-ened, 1 cup	103	0.4	tr.	0	0	0
Rhubarb, stewed and unsweet-ened, 1 cup	12	0	0	0	0	0
Strawberries, 1 cup						
fresh	45	0.2	tr.	0	0	0
frozen, sweetened	245	0.3	tr.	0	0	0
frozen, unsweet-ened	52	0.2	tr.	0	0	0
Sugar apple, 1 medium	146	0.5	tr.	0	0	0
Tangelo, 1 medium	39	0.1	tr.	0	0	0
Tangerine, 1 medium	37	0.2	tr.	0	0	0
Watermelon, 1 cup	50	0.2	tr.	0	0	0

Item and serving	Calories	Total fat (grams)	% total fat	Saturated fat (grams)	% saturated fat	Cholesterol (milligrams)
VEGETABLES						
Alfalfa sprouts, ½ cup	5	0.1	tr.	0	0	0
Artichoke, boiled, 1 medium	53	0.2	tr.	0	0	0
Artichoke hearts, boiled, ½ cup	37	0.1	tr.	0	0	0
Asparagus, ½ cup	22	0.3	tr.	0.1	tr.	0
Bamboo shoots, ½ cup	21	0.2	tr.	0.1	tr.	0
Beans, ½ cup						
all types, cooked without fat	124	0.4	tr.	0.2	tr.	0
baked, brown sugar and molasses	132	1.5	10	0.2	tr.	0
baked w/ham and tomato sauce	123	1.3	9	0.5	tr.	8
baked, vegetarian	235	0.6	tr.	0.3	tr.	0
homestyle, canned	132	0.1	tr.	0.3	tr.	0
Beets, pickled, ½ cup	75	0.1	tr.	0	0	0
Black-eyed peas, ½ cup	99	0.5	tr.	0.1	tr.	0
Broccoli, ½ cup cooked	46	0.4	tr.	0	0	0
frozen w/butter sauce	51	2.3	40	N/A	N/A	N/A
frozen w/cheese sauce	116	6.2	48	1.7	13	5
frozen, chopped	25	0.3	tr.	0.1	tr.	0

Item and serving	Calo-ries	Total fat (grams)	% total fat	Satu-rated fat (grams)	% satu-rated fat	Choles-terol (milli-grams)
VEGETABLES (*cont.*)						
raw	12	0.2	tr.	0	0	
Brussels sprouts, cooked, ½ cup	30	0.3	tr.	0	0	0
Butter beans, ½ cup, canned	100	0.6	tr.	0	0	0
Cabbage, 1 cup						
Chinese, raw	10	0.2	tr.	0	0	0
green, cooked	16	0.1	tr.	0	0	0
red, raw, shredded	10	0.1	tr.	0	0	0
Carrot, 1 large	32	0.2	tr.	0	0	0
cooked, ½ cup	35	0.1	tr.	0	0	0
Cauliflower, 1 cup cooked	30	0.2	tr.	0	0	0
frozen w/cheese sauce	218	12.2	50	N/A	N/A	N/A
raw	12	0.2	tr.	0	0	0
Celery, 1 stalk	6	0.1	tr.	0	0	0
cooked, ½ cup	11	0.1	tr.	0	0	0
Chard, cooked, 1 cup	35	0.2	tr.	0	0	0
Chick peas, 1 cup	268	4.2	14	0.4	tr.	0
Chilies, ¼ cup	14	0	0	0	0	0
Chinese-style fro-zen vegetables, ½ cup	79	4.7	53	0	0	0
Collard greens, 1 cup	26	0.2	tr.	0	0	0
Corn, ½ cup						
canned, cream-style	95	0.4	tr.	0.1	tr.	0

Item and serving	Calo-ries	Total fat (grams)	% total fat	Satu-rated fat (grams)	% satu-rated fat	Choles-terol (milli-grams)
VEGETABLES (*cont.*)						
Corn (*cont.*)						
frozen, cooked	67	0.2	tr.	0	0	0
frozen w/butter sauce	105	2.6	22	N/A	N/A	N/A
canned, whole-kernel	89	1.1	11	0.2	tr.	0
on the cob, 1 me-dium	83	0.9	tr.	0.1	tr.	0
Cucumber, 1 me-dium	16	0.1	tr.	0	0	0
sliced, ½ cup	7	0.1	tr.	0	0	0
Dandelion greens, cooked, ½ cup	17	0.3	tr.	0	0	0
Eggplant, boiled, drained, 1 cup	26	0.2	tr.	0	0	0
Endive, 1 cup	8	0.1	tr.	0	0	0
Green beans, ½ cup						
french-style, cooked	18	0.1	tr.	0	0	0
snap, cooked	22	0.1	tr.	0	0	0
Hominy, white or yellow, cooked, 1 cup	138	0.7	tr.	0	0	0
Italian-style frozen vegetables, ½ cup	130	7.0	48	0	0	0
Kale, cooked, ½ cup	21	0.3	tr.	0	0	0
Kidney beans, 1 cup	224	1.0	4	0	0	0
Leeks, ½ cup						
chopped, raw	32	0.1	tr.	0	0	0

Item and serving	Calo-ries	Total fat (grams)	% total fat	Satu-rated fat (grams)	% satu-rated fat	Choles-terol (milli-grams)
VEGETABLES (cont.)						
chopped, cooked	16	0.1	tr.	0	0	0
Lentils, cooked, 1 cup	232	0.8	tr.	0	0	0
Lettuce, leaf, 1 cup	10	0.2	tr.	0	0	0
Lima beans, 1 cup	216	0.8	tr.	0.1	tr.	0
Mushrooms						
canned, 1 cup	38	0.2	tr.	0	0	0
raw, 1 cup	18	0.2	tr.	0	0	0
fried, 4 medium	78	7.4	85	N/A	N/A	0
Mustard greens, cooked, 1 cup	26	0.8	tr.	0	0	0
Okra, cooked, 1 cup	25	0.1	tr.	0	0	0
Onions						
french-fried, 1 oz.	175	15.0	77	6.9	35	0
raw, chopped, 1 cup	54	0.4	tr.	0	0	0
Parsnips, ½ cup, boiled and drained	63	0.2	tr.	0	0	0
Peas						
canned, ½ cup	61	0.2	tr.	0	0	0
fresh, ½ cup	67	0.3	tr.	0	0	0
frozen, ½ cup	42	0.2	tr.	0	0	0
Pepper, sweet bell						
1 medium	18	0.3	tr.	0	0	0
½ cup, raw	12	0.2	tr.	0	0	0
Pimientos, 1 oz.	10	0	0	0	0	0

Item and serving	Calo-ries	Total fat (grams)	% total fat	Satu-rated fat (grams)	% satu-rated fat	Choles-terol (milli-grams)
VEGETABLES (cont.)						
Potato						
baked w/skin, 1 medium (6 oz.)	220	0.2	tr.	0.1	tr.	0
au gratin, ½ cup						
from a mix, ½ cup	140	6.0	38	3.1	20	6
homemade, ½ cup	160	9.3	52	5.8	32	29
boiled, ½ cup	116	0.1	tr.	0	0	0
french fries, 10						
frozen	111	4.4	36	2.1	17	0
homemade	158	8.3	47	2.5	14	0
hash browns, ½ cup	163	10.9	60	3.4	19	23
knishes, 1 piece	73	3.2	40	0.8	tr.	15
mashed, ½ cup, from flakes	118	5.9	45	3.6	27	15
w/milk and mar-garine	111	4.4	35	1.1	9	2
pancake, 1	495	12.6	23	3.4	6	93
pan-fried, ½ cup	157	12.1	70	1.5	8	7
puffs, frozen, prepared w/oil	183	11.6	57	3.2	16	0
scalloped, ½ cup						
from mix	127	5.9	42	3.6	25	10
homemade	105	4.8	41	2.8	24	14
with cheese	177	9.7	50	N/A	N/A	N/A
twice-baked w/cheese	180	9.9	49	3.3	16	10

Item and serving	Calo-ries	Total fat (grams)	% total fat	Satu-rated fat (grams)	% satu-rated fat	Choles-terol (milli-grams)
VEGETABLES (cont.)						
Pumpkin, canned, 1 cup	82	0.2	tr.	0	0	0
boiled, drained, 1 cup	48	0.1	tr.	0	0	0
Radish, raw, 10	7	0.2	tr.	0	0	0
Sauerkraut, ½ cup	22	0.2	tr.	0	0	0
Scallions, 5 medium	45	0.2	tr.	0	0	0
Snow peas, ½ cup	30	0.3	tr.	0	0	0
Spinach, 1 cup						
cooked	58	0.4	tr.	0.1	tr.	0
creamed	614	11.4	17	1.6	2	1
raw	22	0.2	tr.	0	0	0
Squash, ½ cup						
acorn, baked	57	0.1	tr.	0	0	0
acorn, mashed	41	0.2	tr.	0	0	0
butternut, boiled	41	0.1	tr.	0	0	0
summer, cooked	18	0.3	tr.	0	0	0
raw, sliced	13	0.1	tr.	0	0	0
winter, cooked	39	0.6	tr.	0.1	tr.	0
Succotash, ½ cup	111	0.8	tr.	0.1	tr.	0
Sweet potato						
baked, 1 medium	118	0.1	tr.	0	0	0
candied, ½ cup	192	3.8	18	1.4	6	8
canned in heavy syrup, ½ cup	115	1	8	0.2	tr.	0
mashed, ½ cup	172	0.5	tr.	0	0	0
Tomato						
parboiled, ½ cup	30	0.3	tr.	0	0	0
raw, 1 medium	24	0.3	tr.	0	0	0
stewed, ½ cup	34	0.2	tr.	0	0	0

Item and serving	Calo-ries	Total fat (grams)	% total fat	Satu-rated fat (grams)	% satu-rated fat	Choles-terol (milli-grams)
VEGETABLES (cont.)						
Tomato paste, 1 cup	220	2.4	10	0.4	tr.	0
Turnip greens, 1 cup	30	0.4	tr.	0	0	0
Turnips, ½ cup	14	0.1	tr.	0	0	0
Water chestnuts, canned, sliced, 1 cup	70	0	0	0	0	0
Watercress, ½ cup	2	0	0	0	0	0
Wax beans, ½ cup	25	0.2	tr.	0	0	0
Yam, ½ cup, boiled or baked	79	0.1	tr.	0	0	0
Zucchini, 1 cup	14	0.1	tr.	0	0	0
VEGETABLE SALADS						
Caesar salad w/o anchovies, 1 cup	80	7.2	81	1.5	17	19
Carrot-raisin salad w/mayo, ½ cup	157	3.7	21	1.2	7	49
Chef salad w/o dressing, 1 cup	71	4.3	54	2.0	25	39
Coleslaw, ½ cup mayo-type dress-ing	147	14.2	87	0.2	tr.	5
Gelatin salad, ½ cup, w/fruit and cheese	74	4.6	56	0	0	0
Macaroni salad w/mayo, ½ cup	200	12.8	57	2.5	11	12

Item and serving	Calo-ries	Total fat (grams)	% total fat	Satu-rated fat (grams)	% satu-rated fat	Choles-terol (milli-grams)
VEGETABLE SALADS (cont.)						
Pasta primavera salad, 1 cup	149	5.9	35	0.8	tr.	0
Potato salad						
German, ½ cup	140	3.5	22	N/A	N/A	N/A
w/mayo, ½ cup	189	11.5	55	1.8	8	85
Seven-layer salad, 1 cup	226	17.8	71	6.1	24	105
Tabbouli salad, ½ cup	173	9.5	49	1.4	7	0
Taco salad w/taco sauce, 1 cup	202	14.0	62	6.4	28	41
Three-bean salad, ½ cup	145	11.2	70	1.7	10	0
w/o oil, ½ cup	90	0.3	tr.	0	0	0
Vinaigrette	77	5.5	64	0	0	0
Waldorf salad w/mayo, ½ cup	157	12.7	72	2.8	16	11
GRAINS AND GRAIN PRODUCTS						
Bagel, plain, 3 oz.	163	1.4	7	0.2	tr.	0
Barley flour, 1 cup	698	0.5	tr.	0.3	tr.	0
Biscuit, 1 medium						
baking powder	156	6.6	38	1.9	11	3
buttermilk	103	4.8	42	1.2	10	2
from mix	121	4.3	32	1.2	9	3
Bisquik mix, 1 cup	511	17.0	30	4.1	7	0
Boston brown bread, ½″ slice w/o raisins, canned	85	0.6	tr.	0.2	tr.	N/A

Item and serving	Calo-ries	Total fat (grams)	% total fat	Satu-rated fat (grams)	% satu-rated fat	Choles-terol (milli-grams)
GRAINS AND GRAIN PRODUCTS (cont.)						
Boston brown bread (cont.)						
w/raisins, canned	88	0.6	tr	0.2	tr.	N/A
Bread, 1 slice						
buttermilk	71	1.1	14	N/A	N/A	5
French/Vienna	70	1.0	13	N/A	N/A	0
fruit w/nuts	160	7.0	39	N/A	N/A	N/A
fruit w/o nuts	127	3.4	24	N/A	N/A	N/A
honey wheat-berries	70	1.1	14	N/A	N/A	2
Italian	78	0.5	tr.	N/A	N/A	N/A
"lite" varieties	40	0.5	tr.	0.1	tr.	3
mixed grains	70	0.9	tr.	N/A	N/A	N/A
pita, plain	240	0.8	tr.	N/A	N/A	N/A
pita, whole wheat	236	1.2	5	0.2	tr.	0
raisin	70	1.0	13	N/A	N/A	1
Roman Meal	68	1.0	12	N/A	N/A	5
rye, American	66	0.9	tr	N/A	N/A	N/A
rye, pumper-nickel	82	0.8	tr.	N/A	N/A	N/A
sourdough	68	0.5	tr.	N/A	N/A	0
wheat, commer-cial	61	1.0	14	N/A	N/A	0
white, commer-cial	64	0.9	tr.	N/A	N/A	N/A
white, homemade	72	1.7	21	N/A	N/A	N/A
whole wheat, commercial	61	1.1	16	N/A	N/A	N/A
whole wheat, homemade	67	1.6	21	N/A	N/A	N/A

Item and serving	Calo-ries	Total fat (grams)	% total fat	Satu-rated fat (grams)	% satu-rated fat	Choles-terol (milli-grams)
GRAINS AND GRAIN PRODUCTS (*cont.*)						
Bread crumbs, 1 cup	392	4.6	11	1.1	3	N/A
Breadsticks, 1 piece						
plain	23	0.2	tr.	0.1	tr.	N/A
sesame	56	3.7	60	1.2	19	N/A
soft type, 1 medium	28	0.1	tr.	0	0	N/A
Bulgur, dry, 1 cup	548	2.3	4	N/A	N/A	0
Cereals						
All-Bran, ¾ cup	159	1.1	6	0.2	tr.	0
Alpha-bits, 1 cup	111	0.6	tr.	0.2	tr.	0
Apple Jacks, 1 cup	110	0.1	tr.	0	0	0
bran, 100%, ½ cup	84	1.9	20	0.3	tr.	0
bran, unprocessed, dry, ¼ cup	29	0.6	tr.	0.1	tr.	0
Bran Buds, ⅓ cup	72	0.7	tr.	0.1	tr.	0
Bran Chex, 1 cup	136	1.2	8	0.2	tr.	0
Bran Flakes, 40%, 1 cup	127	0.7	tr.	0.1	tr.	0
Cap'n Crunch, ¾ cup	121	3.4	25	1.7	13	0
Cheerios, 1 cup	90	1.6	16	0.3	tr.	0
Corn Chex, 1 cup	111	0.1	tr.	0	0	0
Cornflakes, 1 cup	108	0.1	tr.	0	0	0
corn grits, w/o added fat, ½ cup	71	0.5	tr.	0	0	0

Item and serving	Calories	Total fat (grams)	% total fat	Saturated fat (grams)	% saturated fat	Cholesterol (milligrams)
GRAINS AND GRAIN PRODUCTS (*cont.*)						
Cereals (*cont.*)						
Cracklin' Oat Bran, ⅓ cup	72	1.3	16	1.3	16	0
Cream of Wheat, w/o added fat, ½ cup	67	0	0	0	0	0
Fiber One, 1 cup	128	2.2	15	0.4	tr.	0
Fruit Loops, 1 cup	111	0	0	0	0	0
Frosted Mini-Wheats, 4 biscuits	102	0.3	tr.	0	0	0
Fruit & Fiber, ½ cup w/apples and cinnamon	90	0.3	tr.	0	0	0
w/dates, raisins, and walnuts	89	0.7	tr.	0.1	tr.	0
Golden Grahams, 1 cup	136	1.1	7	0.1	tr.	0
granola, ⅓ cup, commercial brand	186	6.9	33	3.3	16	0
homemade	184	10.0	49	4.8	23	0
Grapenut Flakes, 1 cup	116	0.4	tr.	0	0	0
Grapenuts, ¼ cup	104	0.2	tr.	0.1	tr.	0
Honeynut Cheerios, ¾ cup	107	0.7	tr.	0.1	tr.	0
Kix, 1½ cup	110	0.7	tr.	0.2	tr.	0
Life, 1 cup	162	2.6	14	0.5	tr.	0

Item and serving	Calo-ries	Total fat (grams)	% total fat	Satu-rated fat (grams)	% satu-rated fat	Choles-terol (milli-grams)
GRAINS AND GRAIN PRODUCTS (cont.)						
Most, ⅔ cup	95	0.3	tr.	0	0	0
Mueslix, Kellogg's, ½ cup	140	1.0	6	0.8	tr.	0
Nutri-Grain, ¾ cup						
barley	106	0.2	tr.	N/A	N/A	0
corn	108	0.7	tr.	N/A	N/A	0
wheat	102	0.3	tr.	N/A	N/A	0
oat bran, cooked, w/o fat, ½ cup	55	1.2	20	0.4	tr.	0
oatmeal, cooked, w/o fat, ½ cup	72	1.2	15	0.2	tr.	0
Product 19, 1 cup	108	0.2	tr.	0	0	0
Puffed Rice, 1 cup	56	0	0	0	0	0
Puffed Wheat, 1 cup	44	0.1	tr.	0	0	0
Raisin Bran, 1 cup	156	0.8	tr.	0.1	tr.	0
Rice Chex, 1 cup	111	0.1	tr.	0	0	0
Rice Crispies, 1 cup	110	0.2	tr.	0	0	0
Shredded Wheat, 1 cup	85	0.5	tr.	0.1	tr.	0
squares, fruit-filled, ½ cup	90	0	0	0	0	0
Special K, 1 cup	111	0.1	tr.	0	0	0
Sugar Frosted Flakes, 1 cup	147	0	0	0	0	0
Sugar Smacks, ¾ cup	106	0.5	tr.	0	0	0
Team, 1 cup	111	0.5	tr.	0.1	tr.	0

Item and serving	Calo-ries	Total fat (grams)	% total fat	Satu-rated fat (grams)	% satu-rated fat	Choles-terol (milli-grams)
GRAINS AND GRAIN PRODUCTS (*cont.*)						
Cereals (*cont.*)						
Total, 1 cup	100	0.7	tr.	0.1	tr.	0
Wheat Chex, 1 cup	169	1.2	6	0.2	tr.	0
Wheat germ, toasted, ¼ cup	108	3.0	25	0.5	tr.	0
Wheaties, 1 cup	99	0.5	tr.	0.1	tr.	0
Coffee cake, 1 piece	233	7.0	27	2.1	8	19
Cornbread, 1 piece						
from mix	160	4.0	22	1.3	7	15
homemade	198	7.3	33	2.2	1	17
Cornmeal, 1 cup	502	1.6	3	0.3	tr.	0
Cornstarch, 1 tbs.	35	0	0	0	0	0
Crackers						
Captain's wafers, 2	30	1.0	3	0.4	tr.	0
cheese, 5	81	4.9	54	1.6	17	4
Cheese Nips, 13	70	3.0	38	1.1	14	3
cheese w/peanut butter, 2 oz.	283	13.5	43	3.0	9	1
Goldfish, 12	34	2.0	21	0.7	tr.	0
graham, 2 squares	60	1.3	19	0.5	tr.	0
Harvest wheat, 4	72	3.6	45	1.1	2	0
Hi Ho, 4	82	4.4	48	1.3	14	1
matzoh, 1 board	115	0.9	tr.	0.2	tr.	0
Melba toast, 1	15	0.2	tr.	0	0	0
Norwegian flat-bread, 2 thin	40	0.3	tr.	0	0	0

Item and serving	Calo-ries	Total fat (grams)	% total fat	Satu-rated fat (grams)	% satu-rated fat	Choles-terol (milli-grams)
GRAINS AND GRAIN PRODUCTS (*cont.*)						
Oyster, 33 pieces	120	3.3	25	0.7	tr.	0
Premium fat-free, 5	50	0	0	0	0	0
rice cake, 1	35	0.3	tr.	0	0	0
rice wafer, 3	31	0	0	0	0	0
Ritz, 3	54	2.9	48	1.1	18	1
Ritz Bits, 22	80	5.0	56	1.6	18	1
Ritz Cheese, 3	70	2.9	37	1.1	14	1
Rye w/cheese, 1.5 oz.	205	9.5	tr.	3.0	13	3
Ryekrisp, plain, 2	50	0.2	tr.	0	0	0
Ryekrisp, ses-ame, 2	60	1.5	22	0.4	tr.	0
Saltines, 2	26	0.6	tr.	0.1	tr.	0
Sesame wafers, 3	70	3.0	38	0.8	tr.	0
Sociables, 6	70	3.0	38	1.1	14	0
soda, 5	42	1.6	34	0.4	tr.	0
Triscuit, 2	42	1.3	28	0.2	tr.	0
Uneeda, 2	42	1.0	21	0.3	tr.	0
Vegetable Thins, 7	70	4.0	51	1.0	13	0
Wasa, 1 piece	45	1.0	21	0.2	tr.	0
Waverly Wafers, 2	36	1.6	40	0.6	tr.	0
Wheat Thins, 4						
regular	36	1.4	35	0.5	tr.	0
nutty	45	2.8	56	0.9	tr.	0
Wheatsworth, 5	70	3.0	38	1.0	13	0
Wheat w/cheese, 1.5 oz.	212	10.9	46	3.0	13	1
Zwieback, 2	40	0.7	tr.	0.2	tr.	0

Item and serving	Calo-ries	Total fat (grams)	% total fat	Satu-rated fat (grams)	% satu-rated fat	Choles-terol (milli-grams)
GRAINS AND GRAIN PRODUCTS (*cont.*)						
Crepe, 1 medium	48	1.5	28	0.5	tr.	37
Croissant, 1 me-dium	167	11.5	62	6.9	37	30
Croutons, ¼ cup	44	1.9	39	1.6	33	0
Danish pastry, 1 medium	256	19.3	68	6.8	24	30
Doughnut, 1 me-dium						
cake	182	7.6	37	3.4	17	27
yeast	239	14.3	54	6.5	24	24
English muffin, 1						
plain	135	1.1	7	0.2	tr.	0
w/raisins	150	1.2	7	0.2	tr.	0
whole wheat	139	2.5	16	0.2	tr.	0
Flour, 1 cup						
carob	452	2.0	4	N/A	N/A	0
rice	428	1.3	3	0.5	tr.	0
rye	308	1.5	4	0.2	tr.	0
soybean	380	18.0	43	2.5	6	0
wheat, cake	349	0.8	tr.	0.1	tr.	0
white, bread	409	1.2	3	0.2	tr.	0
white, all-purpose	418	1.2	2	0.2	tr.	0
white, self-rising	436	1.2	2	0	0	0
whole wheat	399	2.4	5	0	0	0
French toast, 1 slice						
frozen variety	139	6.0	39	1.0	6	54
homemade	172	10.7	56	2.6	14	75
Hushpuppy, 1 me-dium	146	11.4	70	3.0	18	18

Item and serving	Calories	Total fat (grams)	% total fat	Saturated fat (grams)	% saturated fat	Cholesterol (milligrams)
GRAINS AND GRAIN PRODUCTS (cont.)						
Macaroni, 1 cup						
semolina	159	0.7	tr.	0	0	0
whole wheat	183	0.1	tr.	0.1	tr.	0
Matzoh ball, 1	121	7.6	56	2.2	16	76
Muffins, 5 oz.						
banana-nut	135	5.0	33	2.2	15	20
blueberry, from mix	126	4.3	31	1.9	13	9
bran, homemade	112	5.1	41	2.1	17	16
commercial	187	10.3	49	4.3	21	24
corn	130	4.2	29	1.2	8	18
white, plain	118	4.0	30	2.2	17	12
Noodles, 1 cup						
Alfredo	462	29.7	58	9.8	19	73
cellophane, fried	141	4.2	27	0.6	tr.	0
chow mein, canned	306	16.0	47	3.2	9	0
egg	200	2.4	11	0.4	tr.	50
manicotti	129	0.4	tr.	0.1	tr.	0
ramen, all types	188	6.5	32	0.9	tr.	0
rice	140	0	0	0	0	0
Romanoff	372	23.0	56	1.9	29	95
Pancakes, 3 medium						
blueberry, from mix	320	15.0	42	4.3	12	85
buckwheat, from mix	270	12.3	41	3.9	13	90
buttermilk, from mix	270	10.0	33	3.2	11	105

Item and serving	Calo-ries	Total fat (grams)	% total fat	Satu-rated fat (grams)	% satu-rated fat	Choles-terol (milli-grams)
GRAINS AND GRAIN PRODUCTS (*cont.*)						
Pancakes (*cont.*)						
homemade	312	9.6	28	3.0	9	79
"lite," from mix	130	2.0	14	N/A	N/A	10
Popover, 1	170	5.0	26	2.6	14	51
Rice, ½ cup						
brown	116	0.6	tr.	0	0	0
fried	181	7.2	36	0.7	tr.	0
long-grain and wild	120	2.1	16	0.2	tr.	0
pilaf	170	7.0	37	0.6	tr.	0
Spanish-style	106	2.1	18	0.1	tr.	0
white	111	1.2	9	0	0	0
Rice bran, 1 oz.	80	0.4	tr.	0.1	tr.	0
Rolls, 1 small						
Brown & Serve	92	2.2	22	N/A	N/A	5
Cloverleaf	89	3.2	33	0.6	tr.	21
crescent	102	5.6	49	2.8	25	6
croissant	109	6.1	50	3.5	29	21
French	137	0.4	tr.	0.1	tr.	0
hamburger	180	3.0	15	0.8	tr.	1
hard	115	1.2	9	0.3	tr.	1
hot dog	116	2.1	16	0.5	tr.	1
kaiser/hoagie	156	1.6	9	0.4	tr.	2
Parkerhouse	59	2.1	32	0.9	tr.	1
raisin	165	1.7	9	0.4	tr.	0
rye, dark	55	1.6	26	0.1	tr.	0
rye, light, hard	79	1.0	11	0.1	tr.	0
sandwich	162	3.1	17	0.4	tr.	2
sesame seed	59	2.1	32	0.6	tr.	1
submarine	290	3.0	9	0.8	tr.	3
wheat	52	1.7	29	0.4	tr.	0

Item and serving	Calories	Total fat (grams)	% total fat	Saturated fat (grams)	% saturated fat	Cholesterol (milligrams)
GRAINS AND GRAIN PRODUCTS (*cont.*)						
wheat, commercial	110	2.0	16	1.0	8	1
white, homemade	119	3.1	23	0.5	tr.	2
whole wheat	85	1.1	12	0.2	tr.	1
yeast, sweet	198	7.9	36	2.1	9	20
Scone, 1 medium	120	5.5	41	1.5	11	38
Spaghetti, 1 cup	159	1.0	5	0	0	0
Stuffing, ½ cup						
bread, from mix	198	12.2	55	6.0	27	0
cornbread, from mix	175	4.8	25	2.5	13	43
Stove Top	176	9.0	36	5.0	25	21
Sweet roll, iced, 1	198	7.9	41	2.1	9	20
Toaster pastry, any flavor, 1	195	5.0	23	N/A	N/A	N/A
Tortilla, 1 medium						
corn, unfried	48	0.8	tr.	0.1	tr.	0
flour	59	2.5	38	1.1	16	0
Turnover w/fruit, 1	225	19.3	77	N/A	N/A	N/A
Waffle						
frozen, Eggo, 1	120	5.0	37	N/A	N/A	N/A
frozen, other, 1 medium	95	2.6	24	0.7	tr.	11
homemade, 1 large	245	12.6	46	4.1	15	61
MEAT						
Beef, 3 oz., cooked						
Brisket, lean and fat	332	28	76	11	30	79

Item and serving	Calo-ries	Total fat (grams)	% total fat	Satu-rated fat (grams)	% satu-rated fat	Choles-terol (milli-grams)
MEAT (*cont.*)						
Beef (*cont.*)						
Brisket, lean only	205	11	48	4	17	79
Chuck, arm roast						
lean and fat	297	22	66	9	21	84
lean only	196	8	37	3	14	85
Chuck, blade roast						
lean and fat	325	26	72	11	31	87
lean only	230	13	51	5	19	90
Flank, lean and fat	218	13	54	6	16	61
lean only	208	12	52	5	22	60
Ground beef						
extra-lean	213	14	59	5	21	70
lean	227	16	63	6	28	66
regular	244	18	66	7	29	74
Ground, frozen patties (3 oz.)	240	17	64	7	26	80
Rib, large end						
lean and fat	321	27	76	12	34	74
lean only	198	12	55	5	23	70
Rib, small end						
lean and fat	277	21	68	9	29	71
lean only	188	10	48	4	19	68
Rib, short						
lean and fat	400	36	81	15	34	80
lean only	251	15	54	7	25	79
Rib, whole (6–12)						
lean and fat	308	25	73	11	32	73
lean only	194	11	51	5	23	69

Item and serving	Calo-ries	Total fat (grams)	% total fat	Satu-rated fat (grams)	% satu-rated fat	Choles-terol (milli-grams)
MEAT *(cont.)*						
Rib eye, small end						
lean and fat	250	18	65	7	25	70
lean only	191	10	47	4	19	68
Round, bottom						
lean and fat	222	13	52	5	20	81
lean only	189	8	38	3	14	81
Round, eye of						
lean and fat	206	12	52	5	22	62
lean only	155	6	35	2	12	59
Round, full cut						
lean and fat	233	16	62	6	23	71
lean only	165	7	38	2	11	70
Round, tip						
lean and fat	213	13	55	5	22	70
lean only	162	6	33	2	11	69
Round, top						
lean and fat	179	7	35	3	15	72
lean only	162	5	28	2	11	72
Shank crosscuts						
lean and fat	208	10	43	4	17	67
lean only	171	5	26	2	11	66
Short loin, porter-house steak						
lean and fat	254	18	64	7	25	70
lean only	185	9	44	4	19	68
Short loin, T-bone steak						
lean and fat	276	21	68	9	29	71
lean only	182	9	44	4	19	68

Item and serving	Calo-ries	Total fat (grams)	% total fat	Satu-rated fat (grams)	% satu-rated fat	Choles-terol (milli-grams)
MEAT (cont.)						
Beef (cont.)						
Short loin, ten-derloin						
lean and fat	226	15	60	6	24	73
lean only	174	8	41	3	15	72
Short loin, top						
lean and fat	238	16	60	7	26	67
lean only	172	8	42	3	16	65
Wedge-bone sir-loin						
lean and fat	238	15	57	6	23	77
lean only	177	7	35	3	15	76
Variety meats						
brains	167	13	70	3	16	1696
heart	148	5	30	1	6	164
kidneys	122	3	22	1	7	329
liver	137	4	13	2	13	331
lungs	102	3	26	1	9	236
suet, 1 oz.	242	27	100	15	56	19
tongue	241	18	67	8	30	91
tripe, raw, 4 oz.	111	4	32	2	16	107
Beef, cured						
Breakfast strips, cooked, 6 oz.	764	58	68	24	28	202
Corned beef, 3 oz.	213	16	67	5	21	83
Lamb, 3½ oz., cooked						
Blade chop						
lean and fat	380	26	61	15	35	95
lean only	280	12	39	3	9	50

Item and serving	Calo-ries	Total fat (grams)	% total fat	Satu-rated fat (grams)	% satu-rated fat	Choles-terol (milli-grams)
MEAT (*cont.*)						
Leg, lean and fat	242	14	52	9	33	97
lean only	180	8	40	3	15	100
Loin chop, lean and fat	302	22	65	12	36	58
lean only	180	8	40	4	20	80
Rib chop, lean and fat	292	21	65	13	40	70
lean only	180	8	40	5	56	50
Shoulder, lean and fat	430	27	56	15	31	97
lean only	248	10	36	5	18	100
Pork						
Bacon, 1 slice	101	3	27	1	9	5
Bacon bits, 1 tbs.	181	1	5	N/A	N/A	6
Blade, lean and fat, 1 oz.	290	18	56	8	25	67
lean only, 1 oz.	219	9	37	6	16	116
Boston butt						
lean and fat	348	28	72	10	26	88
lean only	304	14	41	5	15	89
Canadian bacon, 1 oz.	43	2	42	0.6	tr.	14
Ham, 3 oz.						
cured, butt						
lean and fat	246	13	47	4	15	60
lean only	159	5	28	2	11	38
cured, canned, 3 oz.	120	5	37	2	15	38
cured, shank						
lean and fat	255	14	49	5	18	60
lean only	176	6	31	3	15	59

Item and serving	Calories	Total fat (grams)	% total fat	Saturated fat (grams)	% saturated fat	Cholesterol (milligrams)
MEAT (cont.)						
Pork (cont.)						
Ham, fresh						
lean and fat	306	18	53	7	20	85
lean only	222	6	24	2	8	40
Ham, smoked	175	11	56	4	21	51
Ham, smoked, 95% lean	144	5	31	2	12	53
Ham loaf, glazed	247	15	55	6	22	116
Loin chop						
lean and fat	314	22	63	9	26	90
lean only	170	8	42	3	16	55
Picnic						
cured, lean	211	10	43	4	17	88
fresh, lean	150	7	42	3	18	75
shoulder, lean	162	5	27	3	16	70
shoulder, marbled	234	14	54	6	23	60
Pig's feet, pickled, 1 oz.	56	4	64	1	16	30
Rib chop, trimmed	209	10	43	4	17	81
Rib roast, trimmed	204	10	43	4	17	83
Sausage						
Brown & Serve, 1 oz.	105	9	77	3	26	24
regular link, 1 oz.	104	5	43	2	17	15
patty, 1	100	8	72	3	27	22
Sirloin, lean	207	10	43	4	17	85
Spareribs, 6 medium	396	35	79	12	27	121

Item and serving	Calories	Total fat (grams)	% total fat	Saturated fat (grams)	% saturated fat	Cholesterol (milligrams)
MEAT (cont.)						
Tenderloin, lean	155	5	29	2	11	78
Top loin chop, trimmed	193	8	37	3	14	79
Top loin roast, trimmed	187	7	33	3	14	77
Processed meats						
Beef, chipped, 2 oz.	114	4	31	1	8	24
Beef jerky, 1 oz.	109	4	33	2	16	30
Bologna, beef/ beef and pork, 1 oz.	85	8	84	3	32	15
Bratwurst						
pork, 2 oz	256	22	77	8	28	51
pork and beef, 2 oz.	226	21	83	7	28	44
Braunschweiger, 1 oz.	102	8	70	3	26	28
Chicken roll, 1 oz.	30	1	30	1	30	10
Corn dog, 1 oz.	330	20	54	N/A	N/A	0
Ham, chopped, 1 oz.	55	2	32	1	16	17
Hot dog, 1						
beef	145	13	80	9	56	27
chicken	116	9	69	3	23	45
turkey	102	8	70	3	26	39
Kielbasa, 1 oz.	80	8	90	2	22	10
Knockwurst, 2 oz.	209	19	82	2	8	36
Liver pâté, 1 oz.	131	12	82	3	20	43

Item and serving	Calo-ries	Total fat (grams)	% total fat	Satu-rated fat (grams)	% satu-rated fat	Choles-terol (milli-grams)
MEAT (cont.)						
Processed meats (cont.)						
Pepperoni, 1 oz.	148	13	79	5	30	N/A
Pork and beef, 1 oz.	100	9	81	3	27	15
Salami, 1 oz.						
cooked	116	10	77	7	54	30
dry/hard	126	10	71	3	21	16
Sausage, 2 oz.						
Italian	216	17	71	6	25	52
Polish	184	16	78	6	20	20
smoked	229	20	78	9	35	48
Vienna, 1 sausage	45	4	80	1	20	8
Spam, 1 oz.	87	7	72	N/A	N/A	N/A
Turkey						
loaf, 1 oz.	43	3	62	1	21	14
breast, 1 oz.	51	2	35	1	17	12
ham, 1 oz.	36	2	50	1	25	18
pastrami, 1 oz.	40	2	45	1	23	15
roll, 1 oz.	72	5	62	1	13	24
salami, 1 oz.	55	4	65	1	16	23
Veal, 3½ oz., cooked						
arm steak						
lean and fat	298	19	57	9	27	80
lean only	180	5	25	3	15	78
Blade						
lean and fat	276	17	55	7	23	100
lean only	228	8	31	4	16	100
Breast, stewed	256	19	66	9	32	100
Chuck, braised	235	13	49	6	23	101
Cutlet						
breaded	319	15	42	N/A	N/A	N/A

Item and serving	Calo-ries	Total fat (grams)	% total fat	Satu-rated fat (grams)	% satu-rated fat	Choles-terol (milli-grams)
MEAT (cont.)						
Flank, medium fat, stewed	390	32	74	16	37	101
Foreshank, me-dium fat, stewed	216	10	42	5	21	101
Loin, broiled	234	13	50	5	19	109
Loin chop						
lean and fat	250	5	18	3	11	95
lean only	149	13	78	7	42	101
Plate, medium fat, stewed	303	21	62	11	33	101
Rib chop						
fat and lean	264	18	62	6	20	100
lean only	125	5	36	3	22	100
Round						
lean and fat	194	13	60	5	23	102
lean only	277	15	49	7	23	101
Rump, marbled, roasted	225	11	44	6	24	101
Sirloin, roasted						
lean	175	3	15	2	10	90
marbled	181	7	35	3	15	108
Sirloin steak roasted						
lean and fat	305	20	59	9	26	100
lean only	204	6	26	2	8	108

SEAFOOD (3½ oz. w/o added fat)

| Abalone, canned | 80 | >1 | tr. | >1 | tr. | 97 |
| Anchovy, canned, 3 | 21 | 1 | 43 | >1 | tr. | 12 |

Item and serving	Calories	Total fat (grams)	% total fat	Saturated fat (grams)	% saturated fat	Cholesterol (milligrams)
SEAFOOD (cont.)						
Anchovy paste, 1 tsp.	14	1	64	N/A	N/A	N/A
Bass						
freshwater	104	3	26	>1	tr.	60
saltwater, black	93	1	12	>1	tr.	50
saltwater, striped	105	3	23	1	8	70
Bluefish						
broiled	117	3	25	1	7	50
fried	205	13	56	3	13	59
Buffalofish	150	4	25	1	6	72
Butterfish						
Gulf	95	3	28	>1	tr.	60
Northern	184	10	49	2	9	49
Northern, fried	275	19	62	3	9	50
Carp	138	6	39	1	6	72
Catfish						
broiled	103	3	26	>1	tr.	60
breaded and fried	226	13	52	3	12	81
Clams, canned, ½ cup	52	1	17	>1	tr.	25
canned, meat only	126	3	21	>1	tr.	57
fresh, raw, 4 large	63	2	28	>1	tr.	29
Cod, canned	85	>1	tr.	>1	tr.	45
cooked	78	>1	tr.	4	46	40
dried, salted	246	2	7	N/A	N/A	129
Crab, canned, ½ cup	86	2	21	N/A	N/A	76
deviled	188	10	48	1	5	40
fried	273	18	59	>1	tr.	N/A
Crab, Alaska King	96	2	18	>1	tr.	53
Crab cake	178	11	56	1	5	100

Item and serving	Calo- ries	Total fat (grams)	% total fat	Satu- rated fat (grams)	% satu- rated fat	Choles- terol (milli- grams)
SEAFOOD (*cont.*)						
Crappie, white	79	1	11	>1	tr.	60
Crayfish, freshwater	72	>1	tr.	>1	tr.	115
Croaker, Atlantic	133	3	20	1	7	60
white	84	1	11	>1	tr.	60
Cusk, steamed	106	>1	tr.	>1	tr.	N/A
Dolphinfish	85	>1	tr.	>1	tr.	72
Eel, American						
cooked	260	18	62	4	14	74
smoked	281	24	77	5	16	60
Fillets, frozen						
batter-dipped, 2	440	31	63	N/A	N/A	N/A
light and crispy, 2	311	23	66	N/A	N/A	N/A
Fish cakes, frozen and fried	242	14	52	4	15	102
Flatfish	79	>1	tr.	>1	tr.	47
Flounder/sole	68	>1	tr.	>1	tr.	30
Gefilte fish	815	2	2	1	1	50
Grouper	87	1	10	>1	tr.	47
Haddock						
cooked	79	>1	tr.	>1	tr.	50
fried	180	10	50	3	15	60
smoked/canned	103	>1	tr.	>1	tr.	68
Halibut	100	1	9	>1	tr.	30
Herring						
canned or smoked	208	14	60	2	8	66
cooked	176	11	56	2	10	70
pickled	223	15	61	2	8	70
Jack mackerel	143	6	38	2	13	75
Kingfish	105	3	26	>1	tr.	68
Lake trout	241	20	75	4	15	74

Item and serving	Calo-ries	Total fat (grams)	% total fat	Satu-rated fat (grams)	% satu-rated fat	Choles-terol (milli-grams)
SEAFOOD (cont.)						
Lobster, Northern						
broiled w/butter, 12 oz.	308	24	70	N/A	N/A	N/A
steamed, 3½ oz.	191	12	57	3	14	65
Mackerel						
Atlantic	159	7	40	2	11	50
Pacific	109	3	25	>1	tr.	70
Muskellunge	109	3	24	>1	tr.	70
Mussels, canned	114	3	24	N/A	N/A	N/A
meat only	95	2	19	1	9	30
Ocean perch, cooked	88	1	10	>1	tr.	40
fried	227	13	51	N/A	N/A	N/A
Octopus	73	>1	tr.	>1	tr.	48
Oysters, canned	76	2	24	1	12	54
fried	239	14	53	3	11	83
raw, 5–8 medium	66	2	27	1	14	54
scalloped, 6 me-dium	356	18	45	N/A	N/A	N/A
Perch, freshwater, yellow	91	1	9	>1	tr.	80
Pickerel	84	>1	tr.	>1	tr.	N/A
Pike						
blue	90	1	10	>1	tr.	75
Northern	88	1	9	>1	tr.	40
Walleye	93	1	10	1	9	80
Pollock, Atlantic	91	1	10	>1	tr.	70
Pompano	166	10	59	5	27	55
Red snapper	93	2	19	1	9	35
Rockfish, steamed	107	3	26	1	8	40
Roughy, orange	124	7	50	>1	tr.	20

Item and serving	Calo-ries	Total fat (grams)	% total fat	Satu-rated fat (grams)	% satu-rated fat	Choles-terol (milli-grams)
SEAFOOD (cont.)						
Salmon, Atlantic	141	6	38	1	6	55
broiled or baked	182	7	69	2	9	50
Salmon, canned						
Chinook	210	14	60	2	8	60
pink	118	5	38	1	7	54
smoked	176	9	46	1	5	35
Sardines, canned						
Atlantic, in soy oil, 2 sardines	50	3	54	>1	tr.	34
Pacific, in tomato sauce, 1 sar-dine	68	5	66	1	13	23
Scallops, cooked	81	1	11	>1	tr.	30
frozen, fried	194	11	51	2	9	55
steamed	112	1	8	>1	tr.	40
Sea bass, white	96	2	19	1	9	40
Shrimp, canned						
dry-packed, 3½ oz.	116	2	15	1	7	155
wet-packed, ½ cup	87	1	10	>1	tr.	125
fried	225	11	44	1	4	120
raw or boiled	91	2	19	1	10	139
Smelt, canned, 4–5	200	14	63	N/A	N/A	N/A
Sole, fillet	68	>1	tr.	>1	tr.	30
Squid, 3 oz.						
fried	149	6	36	N/A	N/A	N/A
raw	110	1	8	>1	tr.	261
Surimi	98	1	10	>1	tr.	30
Sushi or sashimi	144	5	31	1	6	38
Swordfish	118	4	30	1	7	43

Item and serving	Calo-ries	Total fat (grams)	% total fat	Satu-rated fat (grams)	% satu-rated fat	Choles-terol (milli-grams)
SEAFOOD (cont.)						
Trout						
brook	101	2	18	1	9	53
rainbow	195	11	51	1	5	96
Tuna, canned, 6½ oz.						
light, in oil	440	22	45	3	6	35
light, in water	386	2	5	1	2	70
white, in oil	204	20	88	3	13	58
white, in water	237	4	15	2	7	80
Tuna, raw, 3 oz.						
albacore	177	8	41	>1	tr.	70
bluefin	145	4	25	1	6	37
yellowfin	133	3	20	>1	tr.	57
White perch	114	4	32	1	8	65
Yellowtail	138	5	33	1	6	75
POULTRY (3½ oz., no added fat)						
Chicken, breast, ½ breast						
w/skin, fried	236	11	42	3	11	87
w/o skin, fried	179	6	30	2	10	90
w/skin, roasted	193	8	37	3	14	70
w/o skin, roasted	42	3	19	1	6	80
Chicken, fryers						
w/ skin, batter-dipped and fried	289	17	53	3	9	95
w/o skin, fried	237	11	42	1	4	70
w/skin, roasted	239	14	53	4	15	90
w/o skin, roasted	190	7	33	2	9	80

Item and serving	Calo-ries	Total fat (grams)	% total fat	Satu-rated fat (grams)	% satu-rated fat	Choles-terol (milli-grams)
POULTRY (*cont.*)						
giblets, fried	277	14	45	4	13	446
gizzard, sim-mered	153	4	23	2	12	393
heart, simmered	185	8	39	1	5	194
leg, 1 whole						
w/skin, fried	120	9	67	4	30	99
w/skin, roasted	112	6	48	4	32	105
w/o skin, roasted	76	3	35	1	12	41
liver, simmered	157	6	34	2	11	631
roll, light meat	159	7	40	1	6	60
Chicken, stewers						
w/skin	285	19	60	5	16	79
w/o skin	237	12	45	3	11	83
thigh, 1 whole						
w/skin, fried	180	11	55	3	15	60
w/skin, roasted	153	10	58	3	17	58
w/o skin, roasted	109	6	49	2	16	75
wing, 1 whole						
w/skin, fried	121	9	67	2	15	26
w/skin, roasted	99	7	63	2	18	29
Duck						
w/skin, roasted	337	28	75	10	27	84
w/o skin, roasted	201	11	49	4	18	89
Pheasant, w or w/o skin, roasted	211	9	38	3	13	102
Quail, w/o skin	213	9	38	3	13	102
Turkey						
breast, Louis Rich barbecued	135	5	33	1	6	56

Item and serving	Calo-ries	Total fat (grams)	% total fat	Satu-rated fat (grams)	% satu-rated fat	Choles-terol (milli-grams)
POULTRY (*cont.*)						
Turkey (*cont.*)						
oven-roasted	115	3	23	1	8	35
smoked	120	4	30	1	7	45
Dark meat, roasted						
w/skin	221	12	49	4	16	89
w/o skin	187	7	34	2	9	85
Ground	225	14	56	4	16	85
Ham, cured	128	5	35	2	14	62
Light meat, roasted						
w/skin	197	8	36	2	9	76
w/o skin	157	3	17	2	11	69
Loaf, breast meat	110	2	16	>1	tr.	41
Pattied, breaded, and fried	266	17	57	2	7	30
Roll, light meat	147	7	43	2	12	43
Sausage, cooked	50	3	54	2	36	23
Slice, w/gravy, frozen	95	4	38	1	9	26
Wing Drumettes, Louis Rich, smoked	165	7	38	2	11	70
EGGS						
Boiled, poached, 1 large	79	6	68	2	23	213
Fried w/$\frac{1}{2}$ tbs. fat, 1	104	8	69	3	26	246
Omelet, 3 eggs						
cheese (2 oz.)	510	37	65	12	21	480

Item and serving	Calo-ries	Total fat (grams)	% total fat	Satu-rated fat (grams)	% satu-rated fat	Choles-terol (milli-grams)
EGGS (*cont.*)						
plain	271	21	69	5	17	430
Spanish	329	24	65	7	19	530
Scrambled w/milk, 1	99	8	72	3	27	248
Substitute, frozen, 4 oz.						
Egg Beaters	30	0	0	0	0	0
others	96	7	65	1	9	1
White of egg, 1	16	0	0	0	0	0
Yolk of egg, 1	63	6	85	2	29	213
MILK AND DAIRY						
Butter						
solid, 1 tsp.	36	4	100	2	50	11
solid, 1 tbs.	108	12	10	7	58	33
whipped, 1 tsp.	28	3	100	2	64	8
Butter Buds, 2 tbs.	12	0	0	N/A	N/A	0
Buttermilk						
1% fat, 1 cup	99	2	18	1	9	9
dry, 1 tbs.	25	>1	tr.	>1	tr.	5
Chocolate milk						
2%, 1 cup	179	5	25	3	15	17
whole, 1 cup	250	9	32	5	18	30
Cocoa, hot, 1 cup						
w/skim milk	158	2	11	1	6	12
w/whole milk	218	9	37	6	25	33
mix w/water	110	3	24	1	8	5
lo-cal mix, w/water	50	1	18	>1	tr.	2

Item and serving	Calo-ries	Total fat (grams)	% total fat	Satu-rated fat (grams)	% satu-rated fat	Choles-terol (milli-grams)
MILK AND DAIRY (cont.)						
Condensed milk, sweetened, ½ cup	123	11	80	2	15	3
Cream, 1 tbs.						
heavy	52	5	87	3	52	21
light	44	4	8	2	41	17
Evaporated milk						
skim, ½ cup	97	>1	tr.	0	0	0
whole, ½ cup	126	10	71	5	36	27
Low-fat milk						
1%, 1 cup	102	3	26	2	17	10
2%, 1 cup	121	5	37	2	15	18
Malted milk, 1 cup	236	10	38	6	23	37
Malt powder, 1 tbs.	86	2	21	1	10	4
Milkshake, 1 cup						
chocolate, thick	341	17	45	5	13	32
soft serve	218	7	29	2	8	35
vanilla, thick	274	15	49	6	19	37
Ovaltine, w/1%, 1 cup	173	3	16	1	5	33
Powdered milk, ¼ cup						
nonfat	109	>1	tr.	>1	tr.	6
whole	159	8	45	5	28	31
Skim milk, 1 cup	86	>1	tr.	>1	tr.	4
Whole milk, 1 cup	150	8	48	5	30	34
Yogurt, plain, 1 cup						
low-fat	144	4	25	2	12	14
nonfat	127	>	tr.	>1	tr.	4
whole	139	7	45	5	32	29

Item and serving	Calo-ries	Total fat (grams)	% total fat	Satu-rated fat (grams)	% satu-rated fat	Choles-terol (milli-grams)
MILK AND DAIRY (cont.)						
Yogurt, flavored, 1 cup						
vanilla, low-fat	194	3	14	21	9	11
fruit, low-fat	225	3	12	>1	tr.	10
Yogurt, frozen, ½ cup						
low-fat	115	3	23	2	16	10
nonfat	81	>1	tr.	0	0	0
CHEESE (1 oz.)						
Alpine lace						
mozzarella	35	0	0	0	0	5
American	35	0	0	0	0	5
cheddar	35	0	0	0	0	5
American						
processed	106	9	76	6	50	27
reduced-calorie	50	2	36	2	36	12
Blue	100	8	72	5	45	21
Brick	105	8	68	5	43	27
Brie	95	8	76	5	47	28
Caraway	107	8	67	5	42	30
Cheddar						
grated, ¼ cup	114	9	71	6	47	30
sliced, 1 oz.	114	9	71	6	47	30
Cheese fondue, ¼ cup	170	12	63	7	37	37
Cheese food, cold pack, 2 tbs.	94	8	76	4	38	18
Cheese sauce, ¼ cup	132	10	68	N/A	N/A	N/A

Item and serving	Calo-ries	Total fat (grams)	% total fat	Satu-rated fat (grams)	% satu-rated fat	Choles-terol (milli-grams)
CHEESE (*cont.*)						
Cheese spread						
Kraft, 1 oz.	82	6	66	4	44	16
Cheez Whiz	80	6	67	3	33	16
Colby	112	9	72	6	48	27
Cottage cheese, ½ cup						
1% fat	82	1	11	1	10	5
2% fat	101	2	18	1	9	10
creamed	117	5	38	3	23	17
Cream cheese, 2 tbs.						
lite (Neufchâtel)	74	7	85	4	48	20
regular	99	10	91	6	54	31
Weight Watchers	35	2	51	N/A	N/A	N/A
Edam	101	8	71	5	44	25
Feta	75	6	72	4	48	25
Gjetost	132	8	54	5	34	N/A
Gouda	101	8	71	5	44	31
Gruyére	117	7	54	5	38	32
Hot pepper cheese	92	5	49	4	39	18
Jarlsberg	100	7	63	4	36	16
Kraft						
American singles	90	7	70	4	40	25
Free	45	0	0	0	0	5
Light 'n' Lively	70	4	51	2	26	15
Limburger	93	8	77	5	48	26
Monterey Jack	106	8	68	5	42	30
Mozzarella						
part-skim	72	4	50	2	25	16
whole-milk	80	6	67	4	45	22

Item and serving	Calo-ries	Total fat (grams)	% total fat	Satu-rated fat (grams)	% satu-rated fat	Choles-terol (milli-grams)
CHEESE (cont.)						
Muenster	104	8	69	5	43	27
Parmesan						
grated, 1 tbs.	23	1	39	1	39	4
hard, 1 oz.	111	7	56	5	41	19
Pimento cheese spread	106	9	76	6	51	27
Port du Salut	100	8	72	5	45	35
Port wine, cold pack	100	9	81	5	45	35
Provolone	100	8	72	5	45	20
Ricotta						
lite, reduced-fat	109	4	33	N/A	N/A	15
part-skim	171	10	53	6	31	38
whole-milk	216	16	66	10	42	63
Romano	110	8	49	N/A	N/A	29
Roquefort	105	9	77	6	51	26
Smoked cheese product	91	7	69	N/A	N/A	20
Swiss						
processed	95	7	66	3	28	15
sliced	107	8	50	5	42	26
SALAD DRESSINGS						
Blue cheese						
low-calorie, 1 tbs.	11	>1	tr.	0	0	2
regular, 1 tbs.	77	8	93	1	12	0
Buttermilk, from mix, 1 tbs.	58	6	93	1	15	5
Caesar, 1 tbs.	70	7	90	1	13	13

Item and serving	Calo-ries	Total fat (grams)	% total fat	Satu-rated fat (grams)	% satu-rated fat	Choles-terol (milli-grams)
SALAD DRESSINGS (*cont.*)						
French						
creamy, 1 tbs.	70	7	90	1	13	0
low-calorie, 1 tbs.	22	1	41	>1	tr.	1
regular, 1 tbs.	67	6	80	>1	tr.	0
Garlic, from mix, 1 tbs.	83	9	97	1	11	0
Green goddess						
low-calorie, 1 tbs.	27	2	66	>1	tr.	0
regular, 1 tbs.	68	7	92	1	13	0
Honey mustard, 1 tbs.	89	7	71	1	10	0
Italian						
creamy, 1 tbs.	52	5	86	1	17	0
low-calorie, 1 tbs.	16	1	56	>1	tr.	1
regular zesty, from mix, 1 tbs.	85	9	95	1	11	0
Kraft, free, 1 tbs.	20	0	0	0	0	0
Kraft, low-cal, 1 tbs.	25	1	36	0	0	0
Mayonnaise-type,						
low-calorie, 1 tbs.	19	2	95	>1	tr.	2
regular, 1 tbs.	57	5	79	>1	tr.	4
Oil and vinegar, 1 tbs.	69	7	91	2	26	0
Ranch-style, made w/mayo, 1 tbs.	54	6	100	1	16	4
Russian						
low-calorie, 1 tbs.	23	1	39	>1	tr.	1
regular, 1 tbs.	76	7	83	1	12	0

Item and serving	Calo-ries	Total fat (grams)	% total fat	Satu-rated fat (grams)	% satu-rated fat	Choles-terol (milli-grams)
SALAD DRESSINGS (cont.)						
Sesame seed, 1 tbs.	68	7	92	1	13	0
Sweet and sour, 1 tbs.	29	1	31	>1	tr.	0
Thousand Island						
low-calorie, 1 tbs.	24	2	75	>1	tr.	2
regular, 1 tbs.	59	6	92	1	15	0
NUTS AND FATS						
Almond paste, 1 tbs.	80	5	56	>1	tr.	0
Almonds, 12–15	104	9	78	1	8	0
Bacon fat, 1 tbs.	126	14	100	4	28	9
Brazil nuts, 4 me-dium	114	12	95	2	16	0
Cashews, 6–8	94	8	76	1	9	0
Chestnuts, 3 small	66	1	14	0	0	0
Coconut, dried and shredded, ⅓ cup	135	9	60	5	33	0
Hazelnuts, 10–12	106	11	93	1	8	0
Macadamia nuts, roasted, 6 me-dium	117	12	92	2	15	0
Margarine						
liquid, 1 tsp.	36	4	100	>1	tr.	0
solid, 1 tsp.	36	4	100	>1	tr.	0
solid, reduced-calorie, 1 tsp.	18	2	100	>1	tr.	0
Mayonnaise, 1 tbs.						
regular	99	11	100	2	18	8
reduced-calorie	45	5	100	>1	tr.	3

Item and serving	Calo-ries	Total fat (grams)	% total fat	Satu-rated fat (grams)	% satu-rated fat	Choles-terol (milli-grams)
NUTS AND FATS (*cont.*)						
Mixed nuts						
w/peanuts, 8–12	109	10	82	2	16	0
w/o peanuts, 2 tbs.	110	10	82	2	15	0
No-stick spray (PAM), 2-sec-ond spray	8	>1	tr.	>1	tr.	0
Oil, 1 tbs.						
canola	120	14	100	1	7	0
corn	120	14	100	2	15	0
olive	119	14	100	2	14	0
Puritan	124	14	100	2	14	0
safflower	120	14	100	1	7	0
soybean	120	14	100	2	15	0
Peanut butter, 1 tbs.						
creamy	94	8	76	2	19	0
chunky	95	8	75	2	18	0
Peanuts						
chopped, 2 tbs.	104	9	78	1	8	0
honey-roasted, 2 tbs.	112	9	72	1	8	0
in shell, 1 cup	209	18	77	2	8	0
Pecans, 2 tbs.	90	9	90	>1	tr.	0
Pine nuts, 2 tbs.	85	9	95	1	11	0
Pistachios, 2 tbs.	92	8	78	2	19	0
Poppy seeds, 2 tbs.	44	4	82	>1	tr.	0
Pumpkin seeds, 2 tbs.	93	8	77	3	29	0
Sandwich spread (Miracle Whip), 1 tbs.	69	7	91	1	13	6

Item and serving	Calo-ries	Total fat (grams)	% total fat	Satu-rated fat (grams)	% satu-rated fat	Choles-terol (milli-grams)
NUTS AND FATS (cont.)						
Sesame nut mix, 2 tbs.	65	5	69	2	28	0
Sesame seeds, 2 tbs.	94	9	86	1	9	0
Shortening, 1 tbs., vegetable (Crisco)	108	12	100	3	25	0
Sour cream, 1 tbs.						
cultured	26	2	69	1	35	5
half-and-half	20	2	90	1	45	6
imitation	25	2	72	2	72	0
reduced-calorie	15	1	60	>1	tr.	4
Sunflower seeds, 2 tbs.	102	9	79	1	9	0
Trail mix w/seeds, nuts, and carob, 2 tbs.	87	5	52	1	10	0
Walnuts, 2 tbs.	80	8	90	>1	tr.	0
SNACKS						
Bagel chips, 1 oz.	149	9	54	1	6	0
Bugles, 1 oz.	150	8	48	N/A	N/A	N/A
Cheese straws, 4	109	7	58	6	50	N/A
Cheetos, 1 oz.						
Cheese Puff Balls	161	11	61	5	28	14
Cheese Puffs	159	10	57	5	28	14
Corn chips, 1 oz.						
light	144	10	63	>1	tr.	0
regular	155	10	58	1	6	0

Item and serving	Calo-ries	Total fat (grams)	% total fat	Satu-rated fat (grams)	% satu-rated fat	Choles-terol (milli-grams)
SNACKS *(cont.)*						
Corn nuts, ½ cup, all flavors	420	14	30	6	13	0
Cracker Jacks, 1 oz.	114	1	8	0	0	0
Doo-Dads, ½ cup, Nabisco	140	6	38	N/A	N/A	N/A
Party mix w/cereal, nuts, and pret-zels, 1 cup	312	23	66	2	6	4
Popcorn, 1 cup						
air-popped	23	>1	tr.	0	0	0
caramel	140	4	26	2	13	5
microwave, plain	47	3	57	1	19	0
microwave, but-tered	61	5	74	2	29	1
popped w/oil	38	2	47	>1	tr.	0
Pork rinds, 1 oz.	151	9	54	4	24	24
Potato chips, 1 oz.						
plain	159	11	62	3	17	0
barbecue	149	9	54	3	18	0
Light, Pringles	144	8	50	2	13	0
Regular, Pringles	171	13	68	2	11	0
Potato sticks, 1 oz.	152	10	59	2	12	0
Pretzels						
hard, 1 oz.	111	1	8	>1	tr.	0
soft, 1 large	175	>1	tr.	N/A	N/A	0
Tortilla chips, 1 oz.						
Doritos	139	7	45	1	6	0
Tostitos	145	8	49	1	6	0

Item and serving	Calo-ries	Total fat (grams)	% total fat	Satu-rated fat (grams)	% satu-rated fat	Choles-terol (milli-grams)
CANDY						
Butterscotch						
candy, 6 pieces	116	3	23	>1	tr.	0
chips, 1 oz.	234	7	27	N/A	N/A	0
Candied fruit, 1 oz.						
apricot	94	>1	tr.	0	0	0
cherry	96	>1	tr.	0	0	0
citrus peel	90	>1	tr.	0	0	0
figs	84	>1	tr.	0	0	0
Candy bars, 1 oz.						
Almond Joy	136	8	53	5	33	1
Baby Ruth	141	7	45	2	13	1
Bit-O-Honey	121	2	15	N/A	N/A	N/A
Butterfinger	131	6	41	3	21	0
Chunky, milk chocolate	120	4	30	N/A	N/A	N/A
Chunky, original	143	7	44	N/A	N/A	N/A
Golden Almond, Hershey	161	11	61	2	11	5
Heath	142	9	57	4	25	2
Kit Kat, 1.13 oz.	162	8	44	N/A	N/A	0
Krackle	145	8	49	5	31	5
Mars, 1.7 oz.	230	11	43	N/A	N/A	N/A
Milk chocolate						
Hershey	147	9	55	5	31	6
Nestlé	147	9	55	5	31	6
w/almonds	151	10	59	5	30	5
Milky Way	118	4	31	2	15	2
Mounds	131	7	48	5	34	0
Mr. Goodbar	154	11	64	5	29	4
Nestlé's Crunch	160	8	45	4	23	4

Item and serving	Calo-ries	Total fat (grams)	% total fat	Satu-rated fat (grams)	% satu-rated fat	Choles-terol (milli-grams)
CANDY (*cont.*)						
Candy bars (*cont.*)						
Snickers	135	7	46	N/A	N/A	3
Special Dark, Hershey, 1.02 oz.	157	9	51	N/A	N/A	N/A
Three Mus-keteers	140	4	26	2	13	2
Twix	140	7	45	N/A	N/A	N/A
Candy-coated al-monds, 1 oz.	129	5	34	>1	tr.	0
Caramels, 1 oz.						
plain/chocolate w/nuts	120	7	52	3	23	10
plain or choco-late	114	6	47	2	16	9
Carob raisins, 1 oz.	387	14	33	2	5	0
Chocolate chips, 1 cup						
milk chocolate	872	44	45	24	25	0
semisweet	880	48	49	28	29	0
Chocolate-covered cherries, 1 oz.	123	5	36	3	22	1
cream center, 1 oz.	123	5	36	3	22	1
peanuts, 1 oz.	159	12	68	5	28	0
raisins, 1 oz.	120	5	37	3	23	3
Chocolate Kisses, 6	154	9	52	5	29	6
Chocolate Stars, 7	160	8	45	5	28	5
Creme Eggs, 1 oz., Cadbury	136	6	40	N/A	N/A	N/A

Item and serving	Calo-ries	Total fat (grams)	% total fat	Satu-rated fat (grams)	% satu-rated fat	Choles-terol (milli-grams)
CANDY (cont.)						
English toffee, 1 oz.	113	3	24	2	16	5
Fondant, 1 piece	116	>1	tr.	N/A	N/S	N/A
Fudge, 1 oz.						
chocolate	112	3	23	1	8	1
chocolate w/nuts	119	5	38	1	8	1
Good & Plenty, 1 oz.	106	>1	tr.	0	0	0
Gumdrops, 28 pieces	97	>1	tr.	0	0	0
Hard candy, 6 pieces	108	>1	tr.	0	0	0
Jelly beans, 1 oz.	104	0	0	0	0	0
Licorice, 1 oz.	35	>1	tr.	0	0	0
Life Savers, 5 pieces	39	>1	tr.	0	0	0
Malted-milk balls, 1 oz.	137	7	46	4	26	3
M & M's, 1 oz.						
chocolate only	132	6	41	2	14	3
peanut	145	8	50	2	12	4
Marshmallow, 1 large	25	0	0	0	0	0
Mints, 14 pieces	104	>1	tr.	0	0	0
Peanut brittle, 1 oz.	149	8	48	1	6	0
Peanut butter cups, Reese's, 1 oz.	156	9	52	4	23	3
Peppermint Patty, 1	124	5	36	3	22	1
Reese's Pieces, 1.7 oz.	240	13	49	N/A	N/A	N/A

Item and serving	Calo-ries	Total fat (grams)	% total fat	Satu-rated fat (grams)	% satu-rated fat	Choles-terol (milli-grams)
CANDY (*cont.*)						
Saltwater taffy, 1 oz.	99	2	18	>1	tr.	0
Tootsie Roll, 1 oz.	112	2	16	>1	tr.	0
Yogurt raisins, ½ cup	313	14	40	11	32	2
SWEETS						
Apple betty, ½ cup	347	13	34	3	7	0
Baklava, 1 piece	426	29	61	7	15	7
Brownie, 1 small						
butterscotch	52	2	35	>1	tr.	8
chocolate, Little Debbie	109	4	33	N/A	N/A	NA
chocolate, plain	64	3	42	2	28	14
chocolate w/nuts	64	5	70	1	14	N/A
Hostess	151	6	36	N/A	N/A	N/A
Pepperidge Farm	168	9	48	N/A	N/A	N/A
Cake, 1/12 of whole						
angel food	161	>1	tr.	0	0	0
banana, frosted	410	16	35	3	6	60
Black Forest	279	14	45	2	6	57
butter, frosted	380	13	31	2	5	61
carrot, frosted	420	19	41	5	8	66
chocolate, frosted	388	17	39	4	9	87
coconut, frosted	395	18	41	6	14	53
German choco-late, frosted	407	18	40	4	9	82
gingerbread, 2½″ slice	267	3	10	2	7	2
lemon chiffon	190	4	19	>1	tr.	5

Item and serving	Calories	Total fat (grams)	% total fat	Saturated fat (grams)	% saturated fat	Cholesterol (milligrams)
SWEETS (*cont.*)						
lemon, frosted	410	16	35	3	6	61
marble, frosted	408	16	35	3	7	69
pineapple upside-down	236	9	34	2	8	48
pound	200	9	40	4	18	53
pound, Entenmann, fat-free, 1-oz. slice	70	0	0	0	0	0
shortbread w/fruit	344	9	23	2	5	60
spice, frosted	325	11	30	2	5	52
sponge	194	4	18	0	0	137
streusel swirl	260	11	38	2	7	40
white, frosted	369	15	36	4	9	5
yellow, frosted	391	16	37	6	14	55
Cheesecake, ⅛ pie	372	22	53	10	24	36
Cobbler, ½ cup						
w/biscuit top	209	6	26	2	9	2
w/pie-crust top	236	9	34	4	15	5
Cookie, 1						
animal, 15 cookies	120	3	22	1	7	N/A
anise-seed	63	4	57	2	28	8
anisette toast	95	3	28	>1	tr.	21
arrowroot	24	1	37	N/A	N/A	N/A
Bordeaux, Pepperidge Farm	39	2	46	N/A	N/A	N/A
Capri, Pepperidge Farm	82	5	55	N/A	N/A	N/A
chocolate	56	3	48	1	16	6
chocolate chip homemade	68	4	53	2	26	8

Item and serving	Calo- ries	Total fat (grams)	% total fat	Satu- rated fat (grams)	% satu- rated fat	Choles- terol (milli- grams)
SWEETS (*cont.*)						
Cookie (*cont.*)						
Pepperidge Farm	161	7	39	N/A	N/A	N/A
chocolate sand- wich Oreo-type	49	2	37	0	0	0
fig bar	56	1	16	>1	tr.	6
gingersnap	34	2	53	>1	tr.	N/A
graham cracker, chocolate- covered	62	3	43	1	15	N/A
lemon nut, Pep- peridge Farm	168	9	48	N/A	N/A	N/A
Lido, Pepperidge Farm	90	5	50	N/A	N/A	N/A
macaroon	49	1	18	1	18	0
Milano, Pep- peridge Farm	63	4	57	N/A	N/A	N/A
molasses	71	2	25	1	13	N/A
oatmeal	80	3	34	N/A	N/A	0
oatmeal raisin	83	3	32	1	11	N/A
oatmeal, Pep- peridge Farm, 1 large	153	6	35	N/A	N/A	N/A
Orleans, Pep- peridge Farm	31	2	58	N/A	N/A	N/A
peanut butter	72	3	37	1	12	6
Rice Krispie bar	36	1	25	>1	tr.	0
shortbread	42	2	43	>1	tr.	N/A
Social Tea biscuit	22	>1	tr	>1	tr.	N/A
sugar	89	3	30	1	10	N/A

Item and serving	Calories	Total fat (grams)	% total fat	Saturated fat (grams)	% saturated fat	Cholesterol (milligrams)
SWEETS (cont.)						
sugar wafers, 2 small	53	2	34	<1	tr.	N/A
vanilla-creme sandwich	69	3	39	1	13	0
vanilla wafers, 3	51	2	35	1	18	N/A
Cream puff w/custard, 1	245	15	55	4	15	60
Creamsicle, 1 bar	103	3	26	N/A	N/A	0
Cupcake, 1						
chocolate, frosted	159	6	34	2	11	22
yellow, frosted	160	6	34	2	11	23
Custard, baked, ½ cup	148	7	42	3	18	123
Date bar, 1 bar	93	3	29	1	9	2
Dreamsicle, 1	207	6	26	4	17	17
Dumpling, fruit, 1	324	15	42	5	14	8
Éclair, 1 small						
frosted and custard	316	15	43	6	17	N/A
frosted and whipped cream	296	26	79	11	33	N/A
Fruitcake, 1 piece	154	6	35	1	5	11
Fruit ice, ½ cup	123	0	0	0	0	0
Fudgesicle, 1	196	>1	tr.	>1	tr.	3
Gelatin, ½ cup						
low-calorie	8	0	0	0	0	0
regular	70	0	0	0	0	0
Granola bar, 1 bar	141	7	45	2	13	0
Hostess, 1						
Cupcake	206	7	31	4	17	3

Item and serving	Calo-ries	Total fat (grams)	% total fat	Satu-rated fat (grams)	% satu-rated fat	Choles-terol (milli-grams)
SWEETS *(cont.)*						
Hostess *(cont.)*						
Ding Dong	170	9	48	4	21	6
Fruit Snack Pie	403	20	45	7	16	12
Ho Ho	133	7	47	3	20	8
Honey Bun	572	33	52	N/A	N/A	30
Snoball	137	2	13	1	6	1
Twinkie	144	4	25	1	6	8
Ice cream, ½ cup						
chocolate, 10% fat	134	7	47	5	34	30
chocolate, 16% fat	174	12	62	7	36	44
dietetic	134	7	47	4	28	27
imitation, Tofutti	158	8	46	N/A	N/A	0
Simple Pleasures	120	>1	tr.	0	0	10
strawberry, 10% fat	128	6	42	4	28	38
vanilla, 10% fat	134	7	47	5	33	30
vanilla, 16% fat	175	12	62	7	36	44
vanilla, soft-serve	189	11	52	7	33	76
Weight Watchers	81	>1	tr.	>1	tr.	2
Ice cream bar, 1						
chocolate-covered	178	12	61	10	50	23
Toffee Krunch	149	10	60	7	42	9
Ice cream cake roll, 1	159	7	40	4	23	52
Ice cream drum-stick, 1	188	10	48	4	19	14
Ice cream sand-wich, 1	169	6	32	4	21	12

Item and serving	Calo-ries	Total fat (grams)	% total fat	Satu-rated fat (grams)	% satu-rated fat	Choles-terol (milli-grams)
SWEETS (*cont.*)						
Ice milk, ½ cup						
chocolate	91	3	30	2	20	9
soft-serve	112	2	16	1	8	7
strawberry	106	3	25	1	8	7
vanilla	92	3	29	2	19	8
Ladyfinger, 1	79	2	23	>1	tr.	N/A
Lemon bars, 1 bar	70	3	38	>1	tr.	13
Little Debbie						
Devil Square, 1	131	5	34	N/A	N/A	N/A
Dutch Apple Pie, 2 oz.	207	5	22	N/A	N/A	N/A
Fudge Krispie, 2 oz.	256	7	25	N/A	N/A	N/A
Oatmeal Cremes, 2 pieces	332	13	35	N/A	N/A	N/A
Peanut-Butter Bar, 2 bars	265	14	48	N/A	N/A	N/A
Mousse, chocolate, ½ cup	189	16	76	9	43	124
Napoleon, 1 piece	85	5	53	3	32	10
Pie, ⅛ of whole						
apple	347	17	44	2	5	3
banana cream	353	14	36	10	25	35
blueberry	387	17	40	4	9	N/A
Boston cream	260	8	21	3	10	20
cherry	418	18	39	5	11	N/A
chocolate cream	311	13	38	5	14	15
chocolate me-ringue	378	18	43	7	17	N/A
coconut cream	365	19	47	7	17	N/A

Item and serving	Calo-ries	Total fat (grams)	% total fat	Satu-rated fat (grams)	% satu-rated fat	Choles-terol (milli-grams)
SWEETS (cont.)						
Pie (cont.)						
key lime	388	19	44	7	16	10
lemon chiffon	335	14	38	4	11	N/A
lemon meringue	350	13	33	5	13	8
mincemeat	434	18	37	5	10	N/A
peach	421	18	38	5	11	3
pecan	510	23	41	4	7	N/A
pumpkin	367	17	42	6	15	109
raisin	325	13	36	3	8	N/A
rhubarb	405	17	38	5	11	2
strawberry	228	9	36	5	20	2
sweet potato	342	18	47	6	16	70
Popsicle, 1 bar	96	0	0	0	0	0
Pudding, ½ cup						
bread	219	8	33	3	12	78
chocolate w/whole milk	247	9	33	5	18	47
chocolate, D-Zerta	65	>1	tr.	>1	tr.	2
from mix w/skim milk	124	0	0	0	0	0
noodle	141	5	32	1	6	72
rice	181	6	30	2	9	98
tapioca	126	5	36	2	14	82
vanilla	168	6	32	3	16	70
Pudding Pop, frozen, 1	75	2	24	1	12	2
Sherbet, ½ cup	135	2	13	1	6	7
Sopaipilla, 1 piece	88	6	61	1	10	0

Item and serving	Calories	Total fat (grams)	% total fat	Saturated fat (grams)	% saturated fat	Cholesterol (milligrams)
SWEETS (cont.)						
Soufflé, chocolate, ½ cup	63	4	57	1	14	42
Strudel, fruit, ½ cup	47	1	19	>1	tr.	2
Tart, fruit, 1 small	362	18	45	N/A	N/A	N/A
Tasty Kake, 1						
Butterscotch Krimpet	118	2	15	1	8	7
Chocolate Junior	306	12	35	4	12	4
Coconut Cream	482	31	58	10	19	39
Fruit Pie	362	14	35	5	12	48
Jelly Krimpet	96	1	9	>1	tr.	3
Toppings, 3 tbs.						
caramel	156	>1	tr.	0	0	0
cherry	147	>1	tr.	0	0	0
chocolate fudge	97	4	37	2	19	0
chocolate syrup	73	>1	tr.	>1	tr.	0
custard sauce	64	3	42	1	14	59
lemon sauce	100	2	18	>1	tr.	10
marshmallow creme	158	0	0	0	0	0
milk chocolate fudge, 2 tbs.	124	5	36	3	22	N/A
pecans in syrup	168	3	16	1	5	0
pineapple	146	>1	tr.	0	0	0
raisin sauce	126	3	21	1	7	0
strawberry	139	>1	tr.	0	0	0
Toppings whipped aerosol, ¼ cup	46	4	78	1	20	N/A

Item and serving	Calo-ries	Total fat (grams)	% total fat	Satu-rated fat (grams)	% satu-rated fat	Choles-terol (milli-grams)
SWEETS (*cont.*)						
Toppings (*cont.*)						
from mix, ¼ cup	32	2	56	1	28	4
frozen, ¼ cup	59	5	76	4	61	0
whipping cream						
heavy, 1 tbs.	54	6	100	4	66	21
light, 1 tbs.	45	5	100	3	60	17
Trifle, ½ cup	289	20	62	9	28	88
Turnover w/fruit, 1	226	19	76	5	20	2
Yogurt, frozen						
low-fat, ½ cup	115	3	23	2	16	10
nonfat, ½ cup	81	>1	tr.	0	0	0
BEVERAGES						
Apple juice	92	0	0	0	0	0
Beer						
regular	148	0	0	0	0	0
light	100	0	0	0	0	0
low-alcohol	112	0	0	0	0	0
Carbonated drink						
regular	152	0	0	0	0	0
sugar-free	1	0	0	0	0	0
Club soda/seltzer	0	0	0	0	0	0
Coffee, brewed or instant	4	0	0	0	0	0
Coffee, flavored mixes, instant	55	2	33	1	16	0
Cordials and li-queurs, 54 proof	97	0	0	0	0	0

Item and serving	Calo-ries	Total fat (grams)	% total fat	Satu-rated fat (grams)	% satu-rated fat	Choles-terol (milli-grams)
BEVERAGES (*cont.*)						
Daiquiri	122	0	0	0	0	0
Eggnog, non-alcoholic	342	19	50	11	29	149
Gatorade	60	0	0	0	0	0
Gin	39	0	0	0	0	0
Grape juice drink, canned	89	0	0	0	0	0
Hawaiian punch	120	0	0	0	0	0
Kool-Aid, from mix	95	0	0	0	0	0
Lemonade, mix or frozen	102	0	0	0	0	0
Orange juice, un-sweetened	83	0	0	0	0	0
Pineapple-orange juice	99	0	0	0	0	0
Rum	70	0	0	0	0	0
Tang, orange or grape	117	0	0	0	0	0
Tea, brewed or in-stant	0	0	0	0	0	0
Vodka	70	0	0	0	0	0
Whiskey	70	0	0	0	0	0
Wine						
dessert, aperitif	184	0	0	0	0	0
table	83	0	0	0	0	0
wine cooler	83	0	0	0	0	0
FRUIT JUICE AND NECTARS						
Apple juice	116	>1	tr.	0	0	0

Item and serving	Calo-ries	Total fat (grams)	% total fat	Satu-rated fat (grams)	% satu-rated fat	Choles-terol (milli-grams)
FRUIT JUICE AND NECTARS (cont.)						
Apricot nectar	141	>1	tr.	0	0	0
Carrot juice	96	>1	tr.	0	0	0
Cranberry-apple juice	129	>1	tr.	>1	tr.	0
Cranberry juice cocktail						
low-cal	45	0	0	0	0	0
regular	147	>1	tr.	0	0	0
Grapefruit juice	96	>1	tr.	0	0	0
Grape juice	155	>1	tr.	>1	tr.	0
Lemon juice	8	0	0	0	0	0
Lime juice	8	0	0	0	0	0
Orange-grapefruit juice	107	>1	tr.	0	0	0
Orange juice	111	>1	tr.	>1	tr.	0
Peach juice or nec-tar	134	>1	tr.	0	0	0
Pear juice or nectar	149	0	0	0	0	0
Pineapple juice	139	>1	tr.	0	0	0
Pineapple-orange juice	125	1	7	0	0	0
Prune juice	181	1	5	0	0	0
Tomato juice	41	2	44	0	0	0
V8 juice	53	1	17	0	0	0
COMBINATION DISHES						
Baked beans w/pork, ½ cup	134	2	13	1	7	81
Beans and franks, canned, 1 cup	366	16	39	6	15	5

Item and serving	Calo-ries	Total fat (grams)	% total fat	Satu-rated fat (grams)	% satu-rated fat	Choles-terol (milli-grams)
COMBINATION DISHES (*cont.*)						
Beans, refried, ½ cup						
canned	135	1	6	>1	tr.	0
with fat	271	13	43	5	17	12
w/sausage, canned	194	13	60	6	28	25
Beef burgundy, 1 cup	336	21	56	8	21	72
Beef, chipped						
cream, ½ cup	175	11	57	4	21	21
cream, frozen, 5½ oz.	235	16	61	N/A	N/A	N/A
Beef noodle casse-role, 1 cup	329	19	52	6	16	81
Beef Oriental, Lean Cuisine, 9⅛ oz.	270	9	30	N/A	N/A	N/A
Beef pie, 8 oz.						
frozen	430	23	48	6	13	41
homemade	515	30	52	8	14	42
Beef short ribs with gravy, frozen, 5¾ oz.	350	25	64	N/A	N/A	59
Beef sloppy joe, 5 oz.	199	12	54	N/A	N/A	N/A
Beef stew, frozen, 1 cup	184	8	39	N/A	N/A	N/A
Beef Teriyaki, Stouffer's, 10 oz.	365	11	27	N/A	N/A	N/A
Beef vegetable stew, 1 cup	218	11	45	5	21	N/A

Item and serving	Calo-ries	Total fat (grams)	% total fat	Satu-rated fat (grams)	% satu-rated fat	Choles-terol (milli-grams)
COMBINATION DISHES (*cont.*)						
Beef vegetable stew, home-made, 1 cup	244	14	52	5	18	46
Burrito, 1 large						
bean w/cheese	230	10	39	5	20	26
bean w/o cheese	142	3	19	1	N/A	3
beef	424	25	53	10	21	86
with guacamole	354	16	41	N/A	N/A	N/A
Cabbage with ground beef and rice, 1 med.	172	8	42	3	16	26
Cannelloni w/meat and cheese, 1 piece	420	30	64	14	30	185
Cheese soufflé, 1 cup	174	11	57	3	16	132
Chicken à la king						
Stouffer's, 9½ oz.	330	11	30	N/A	N/A	N/A
Swanson, 5¼ oz.	180	12	60	N/A	N/A	N/A
homemade, 1 cup	318	18	51	5	14	67
Chicken and dump-lings, breast and 1 dump-ling	298	11	33	3	9	103
Chicken and Noo-dles, Stouffer's, 5¾ oz.	250	15	54	3	11	55
Chicken and vege-table stirfry, 1 cup	142	7	44	1	6	26

Item and serving	Calories	Total fat (grams)	% total fat	Saturated fat (grams)	% saturated fat	Cholesterol (milligrams)
COMBINATION DISHES (*cont.*)						
Chicken Cacciatore, Stouffer's, 11¼ oz.	310	11	32	N/A	N/A	N/A
Chicken Divan, Stouffer's, 8½ oz.	335	22	59	N/A	N/A	N/A
Chicken fricassee, homemade, 1 cup	328	21	58	7	19	N/A
Chicken-fried steak, 3½ oz.	355	23	58	7	18	115
Chicken, Glazed, Lean Cuisine, 8½ oz.	270	7	23	N/A	N/A	55
Chicken Paprikash, Stouffer's, 10½ oz.	390	15	35	N/A	N/A	N/A
Chicken parmigiana, homemade, 7 oz.	308	15	44	5	15	11
Chicken pot pie, 8 oz.						
frozen	430	23	48	7	15	40
homemade	546	31	51	10	16	56
Chicken salad with mayo, ½ cup	271	21	70	9	30	56
Chicken with almonds, Chinese, 1 cup	203	11	49	2	9	22
Chili, 1 cup						
with beans	302	15	45	6	18	52
without beans	302	19	57	8	24	70

Item and serving	Calories	Total fat (grams)	% total fat	Saturated fat (grams)	% saturated fat	Cholesterol (milligrams)
COMBINATION DISHES (*cont.*)						
Chitterlings, 3½ oz.	303	29	86	10	30	143
Chop suey, 1 cup						
beef, no rice	300	17	51	8	24	N/A
chicken, no rice	124	7	51	1	7	8
fish, no rice	120	6	45	2	15	10
Chow mein, 1 cup						
beef, La Choy	72	2	25	N/A	N/A	N/A
chicken, La Choy	68	2	26	N/A	N/A	N/A
homemade	224	9	36	2	8	N/A
pepper, La Choy	89	1	10	N/A	N/A	N/A
Corned beef hash, 1 cup	374	24	58	7	17	80
Curry, meatless, 1 cup	138	7	46	3	20	15
Deviled crab, ½ cup	231	15	58	4	16	50
Deviled egg, 1 large	63	5	71	1	14	109
Egg foo yung, 1 piece	129	12	84	3	21	107
Eggplant parmesan, 1 cup	356	24	61	9	23	31
Egg roll, frozen, La Choy, 4	112	5	40	N/A	N/A	N/A
Egg salad w/mayo, 1 cup	424	35	74	8	17	654
Enchilada, 1						
bean, beef, and cheese	243	14	52	7	26	38
beef, frozen	250	16	58	N/A	N/A	N/A
cheese, frozen	366	21	52	N/A	N/A	N/A

Item and serving	Calo-ries	Total fat (grams)	% total fat	Satu-rated fat (grams)	% satu-rated fat	Choles-terol (milli-grams)
COMBINATION DISHES (*cont.*)						
chicken, frozen	247	11	40	N/A	N/A	N/A
Falafel, 1 small	74	5	61	1	12	9
Fettucine Alfredo, 1 cup	461	30	59	N/A	N/A	N/A
Fillet of fish divan, frozen, 12⅜ oz.	240	3	11	N/A	N/A	85
Fish creole, 1 cup	172	5	26	N/A	N/A	N/A
Fritter, corn, 1 medium	132	9	61	2	14	0
Frozen dinners						
chopped beef-steak	443	27	55	N/A	N/A	N/A
chopped steak	730	41	51	N/A	N/A	N/A
fried chicken	590	31	47	N/A	N/A	N/A
meat loaf	530	29	49	N/A	N/A	N/A
salisbury steak	500	29	52	N/A	N/A	N/A
turkey	360	11	28	N/A	N/A	N/A
Green pepper stuffed, with ground beef and rice, 1 medium	262	14	48	6	21	52
Hamburger Helper, all varieties, 1 cup	375	19	46	7	17	76
Ham salad w/mayo, ½ cup	277	20	65	4	13	54
Ham spread, Spreadables, ½ cup	271	20	66	10	33	45

Item and serving	Calo-ries	Total fat (grams)	% total fat	Satu-rated fat (grams)	% satu-rated fat	Choles-terol (milli-grams)
COMBINATION DISHES (cont.)						
Lasagna						
cheese, frozen, 10 oz.	385	14	33	N/A	N/A	N/A
homemade with beef and cheese, 8 oz.	400	20	45	10	23	81
Zucchini, Lean Cuisine, 11 oz.	260	6	21	N/A	N/A	N/A
Lobster						
Cantonese, 1 cup	334	20	54	6	16	240
Newburg, 1 cup	388	21	49	N/A	N/A	N/A
salad w/mayo, 1 cup	238	15	57	3	11	136
Lo mein, 1 cup	185	7	34	1	5	11
Macaroni and cheese						
from mix, 1 cup	386	17	40	N/A	N/A	22
frozen, 6 oz.	260	12	42	N/A	N/A	17
Manicotti, cheese and tomato, 1 piece	238	12	45	6	23	61
Meatball with regular ground beef, 1 medium	72	5	62	2	25	30
Meat loaf with regular ground beef, 2½ oz.	237	15	57	6	23	73
Moo goo gai pan, 1 cup	304	17	50	3	6	66

Item and serving	Calories	Total fat (grams)	% total fat	Saturated fat (grams)	% saturated fat	Cholesterol (milligrams)
COMBINATION DISHES (cont.)						
Onion rings, 10	234	17	65	6	23	0
Pepper steak w/ trimmed sirloin, 3 oz.	213	9	38	N/A	N/A	35
Pizza, frozen						
cheese on french bread, 5¼ oz.	330	13	35	7	19	37
pepperoni, frozen, ¼ pizza	364	18	45	9	22	47
Pizza rolls, Jeno, 3	129	7	49	2	14	10
Pork, sweet and sour, 1½ cup	386	22	51	N/A	N/A	80
Quiche, 1 small slice						
Lorraine	360	21	53	N/A	N/A	140
vegetable	312	18	52	N/A	N/A	135
Ratatouille, ½ cup	87	8	83	N/A	N/A	0
Ravioli, canned, 1 cup	240	7	26	4	15	20
Ravioli w/meat and tomato sauce, 1 piece	49	3	55	1	18	19
Salisbury steak w/gravy, 8 oz.	364	27	67	12	30	126
Salmon patty, 3½ oz.	239	12	45	4	15	94
Shepherd's pie, 1 cup	407	24	53	8	18	41
Shrimp creole w/o rice, 1 cup	146	6	37	1	6	123
Shrimp salad w/mayo, ½ cup	136	10	66	2	13	69

Item and serving	Calo-ries	Total fat (grams)	% total fat	Satu-rated fat (grams)	% satu-rated fat	Choles-terol (milli-grams)
COMBINATION DISHES (*cont.*)						
Spaghetti, 1 cup						
w/meat sauce	317	17	48	N/A	N/A	56
w/tomato sauce	179	2	10	>1	tr.	5
Spaghettios, Franco-Ameri-can, 1 cup	160	2	11	N/A	N/A	N/A
Spanakopita, 1 piece	259	24	83	7	24	79
Spinach soufflé, 1 cup	212	15	64	7	30	184
Stroganoff, 1 cup						
beef, Stouffer's	390	20	46	N/A	N/A	72
homemade w/o noodles	568	44	70	19	30	8
Taco, beef, 1 medium	272	17	56	9	29	54
Tamale w/sauce, 1	114	6	47	2	16	3
Tortellini, 1 cup						
meat	363	15	37	5	12	238
cheese	335	14	38	4	11	20
Tostada w/refried beans, 1 medium	294	16	49	7	21	20
Tuna casserole, 1 cup	315	13	37	3	8	38
Tuna Helper, 1 cup	295	10	31	2	6	30
Tuna salad, ½ cup						
oil pack, w/mayo	226	16	64	3	12	20
water pack, w/mayo	170	11	58	2	11	14
Veal parmigian homemade, 1 cup	485	26	48	9	17	102

Item and serving	Calo-ries	Total fat (grams)	% total fat	Satu-rated fat (grams)	% satu-rated fat	Choles-terol (milli-grams)
COMBINATION DISHES (*cont.*)						
frozen, 5 oz.	287	16	50	N/A	N/A	67
Veal scaloppine, 1 cup	429	20	42	9	15	132
Welsh rarebit, 1 cup	415	32	69	17	36	N/A
Wonton w/pork, fried, 1 piece	82	4	44	1	11	21
ODDS AND ENDS						
Bouillon cube, beef or chicken	8	>1	tr.	>1	tr.	0
Chewing gum, 1 stick	10	0	0	0	0	0
Chocolate, baking, 1 oz.	143	15	94	9	57	0
Jam, all types, 1 tbs.	54	0	0	0	0	0
Jelly, all types, 1 tbs.	49	0	0	0	0	0
Marmalade, 1 tbs.	51	0	0	0	0	0
Sugar, all types, 1 tbs.	46	0	0	0	0	0
Syrup, all types, 1 tbs.	60	0	0	0	0	0

HIGH-FIBER FOODS

Apple	Bran muffin	Chick peas
Banana	Brown rice	Chinese cabbage
Barley	Brussel sprouts	Corn on the cob
Berries	Carrots	Dry beans

HIGH-FIBER FOODS (*cont.*)

Figs	Parsnips	Pumpkin
Greens	Pears	Winter squash
Lima beans	Peas	Whole wheat bread
Millet	Plantain	Whole wheat pasta
Papaya	Prunes	

You can easily increase your child's intake of fiber by substituting whole fruits for juices; fruit and vegetables are a good-tasting, natural source of dietary fiber. A diet rich in legumes and peas, such as black beans, navy beans, kidney beans, and split and black-eyed peas (which make great hearty soups and chilis), will also increase your family's fiber intake. Finally, remember to choose whole grain breads and cereals.

Fast-Food
Restaurant Menus

This section is devoted to the menus of a sampling of fast-food restaurants. The lists have been taken from materials supplied by the restaurants themselves and are as complete as we could make them.

A quick survey of the percentage of fat content of the offerings may give you the chills, but referring to the tables will give you a better chance to make intelligent choices — either at home before you go, or sitting down at the restaurant and studying the lists as you would menus. It should be a whole lot easier than trying to choose at the counter with a line of other customers behind you. Even more absurd would be trying to use their eye-straining charts, which are usually hung on a wall far from the counter.

Most of these restaurants are making new additions to their selections, some of which are fat-lowering. These may not be included in our tables as we go to press. Watch for them.

Item	Calories	Total fat (grams)	% total fat	Cholesterol (milli-grams)
ARBY'S				
Roast beef, regular	350	15	39	39
Roast beef, junior	218	8	33	20
Roast beef, super	501	22	40	40
Roast beef, deluxe	486	23	43	59
Beef 'n' cheddar	490	21	39	51
Chicken breast sandwich	592	27	41	57
Potato cakes, 2	201	14	63	1.3
French fries	211	8	34	6
King roast beef	467	19	37	49
Bac 'n' cheddar deluxe	561	34	55	78
Hot ham 'n' cheese	353	13	33	50
Turkey deluxe	375	17	41	39
Baked potato, plain	290	0.05	trace	0
Superstuffed potato, deluxe	648	38	53	72
Broccoli and cheddar	541	22	37	24
Mushroom and cheese	506	22	39	21
Taco	619	27	39	145
Vanilla shake	295	10	31	30
Chocolate shake	384	11	26	32
Jamocha shake	424	10	21	31
Roasted chicken breast	254	7	25	200
Roasted chicken leg	319	16	45	214
Chicken salad sandwich	386	20	47	30
Chicken salad and croissant	472	36	69	12
Chicken salad w/tomato, lettuce	515	36	63	12
Chicken club sandwich	621	32	46	108
Rice pilaf	123	2	15	0
Scandinavian vegetables, sauce	56	2	32	0
Tossed salad, plain	44	0.7	tr.	0

Item	Calories	Total fat (grams)	% total fat	Cholesterol (milli-grams)
ARBY'S *(cont.)*				
Tossed salad w/20-calorie Italian dressing	57	0.9	tr.	0
BURGER KING				
Whopper sandwich	640	41	58	94
Whopper w/cheese	723	48	60	117
Double beef whopper	850	52	55	—
Double beef whopper w/cheese	950	60	57	—
Whopper junior	370	17	41	41
Whopper junior w/cheese	420	20	43	52
Hamburger	275	12	39	37
Cheeseburger	317	15	43	48
Bacon double cheeseburger	510	31	55	104
French fries, regular	227	13	52	14
Onion rings, regular	274	16	52	0
Apple pie	305	12	35	4
Chocolate shake, medium	320	12	36	—
Vanilla shake, medium	321	10	28	—
Vanilla shake, added syrup	334	10	27	—
Chocolate shake, added syrup	374	11	26	—
Whaler fish sandwich	488	27	50	84
Whaler w/cheese	530	30	51	95
Ham and cheese	471	23	44	70
Chicken sandwich	688	40	52	82
Chicken tenders	204	10	44	47
Breakfast croissantwich				
bacon, egg, cheese	355	24	61	249
sausage, egg, cheese	538	41	69	293

Item	Calories	Total fat (grams)	% total fat	Cholesterol (milli- grams)
BURGER KING (*cont.*)				
Breakfast croissantwich (*cont.*)				
ham, egg, cheese	335	20	54	262
Scrambled egg platter	468	30	57	370
w/sausage	702	52	66	420
w/bacon	536	36	60	378
French toast platter				
w/bacon	469	30	57	73
w/sausage	635	46	65	115
Salad, plain	28	0	0	0
w/house dressing	159	13	73	11
w/bleu cheese	184	16	78	22
w/1000 island	145	12	74	17
w/french	152	11	65	0
w/golden Italian	162	14	77	0
w/creamy Italian	—	—	—	—
w/reduced-calorie Italian	42	1	21	0
Cherry pie	357	13	33	6
Pecan pie	459	20	39	4
CHURCH'S				
Fried chicken				
breast	278	17	55	—
wing–breast cut	303	20	59	—
thigh	306	22	65	—
leg	147	9	55	—
Crispy nuggets				
regular	55	3	49	—
spicy	52	3	47	—
Southern-fried catfish	67	4	54	—

Item	Calories	Total fat (grams)	% total fat	Cholesterol (milli-grams)
CHURCH'S (cont.)				
Hush puppies	78	3	35	—
Dinner roll	83	2	22	—
French fries	256	13	46	—
Corn on the cob (buttered)	165	3	16	—
Jalapeño pepper	4	0	0	—
Pecan pie	367	20	49	—
Cole slaw	83	7	76	—
DAIRY QUEEN				
Cone, small	140	4	26	10
Cone, regular	240	7	26	15
Cone, large	340	10	26	25
Dipped cone, small	190	9	43	10
Dipped cone, regular	340	16	42	20
Dipped cone, large	510	24	42	30
Sundae, small	190	4	19	10
Sundae, regular	310	8	23	20
Sundae, large	440	10	20	30
Shake, small	490	13	24	35
Shake, regular	710	19	24	50
Shake, large	990	26	24	70
Malt, small	520	13	23	35
Malt, regular	760	18	21	50
Malt, large	1060	25	21	70
Float	410	7	15	20
Banana split	540	11	18	30
Parfait	430	8	17	30
Peanut butter parfait	740	34	41	30
Double delight	490	20	37	25

Item	Calories	Total fat (grams)	% total fat	Cholesterol (milli-grams)
DAIRY QUEEN (cont.)				
Hot fudge brownie delight	600	25	38	20
Strawberry shortcake	540	11	18	25
Freeze	500	12	22	30
Mr. Misty, small	190	0	0	0
Mr. Misty, regular	250	0	0	0
Mr. Misty, large	340	0	0	0
Mr. Misty Kiss	70	0	0	0
Mr. Misty Freeze	500	12	22	30
Mr. Misty Float	390	7	16	20
Buster bar	460	29	57	10
Dilly bar	210	13	56	10
DQ sandwich	140	4	26	5
Single hamburger	360	16	40	45
Double hamburger	530	28	48	85
Triple hamburger	710	45	57	135
Single w/cheese	410	20	44	50
Double w/cheese	650	37	51	95
Triple w/cheese	820	50	55	145
Hot dog	280	16	51	45
Hot dog w/chili	320	20	56	55
Hot dog w/cheese	330	211	57	55
Super hot dog	520	27	47	80
Super hot dog w/chili	570	32	51	100
Super hot dog w/cheese	580	34	53	100
Fish filet sandwich	400	17	38	50
Fish filet sandwich w/cheese	440	21	43	60
Chicken sandwich	670	41	55	75
French fries, small	200	10	45	10
French fries, large	320	16	45	15
Onion rings	280	16	51	15

Item	Calories	Total fat (grams)	% total fat	Cholesterol (milli-grams)
HARDEE'S				
Hamburger	305	13	38	—
Cheeseburger	335	17	46	—
Big deluxe	546	26	43	77
¼-pound cheeseburger	506	26	46	61
Roast beef sandwich	377	17	41	57
Big roast beef	418	19	41	60
Hot dog	346	22	57	42
Hot ham and cheese	376	15	36	59
Fisherman's fillet sandwich	514	26	46	41
Chicken fillet	510	26	46	57
Bacon cheeseburger	686	42	55	295
Sausage biscuit	413	26	57	29
Sausage egg biscuit	521	35	60	293
Steak biscuit	419	23	49	34
Steak and egg biscuit	527	31	53	298
Ham biscuit	349	17	44	29
Ham and egg biscuit	458	26	51	293
Bacon egg biscuit	405	26	58	305
French fries, small	239	13	49	4
French fries, large	381	21	50	6
Apple turnover	282	14	45	5
Milkshake	391	10	23	42
JACK IN THE BOX				
Hamburger	276	12	39	29
Cheeseburger	323	15	42	42
Jumbo Jack	485	26	48	64
Jumbo Jack w/cheese	630	35	50	110
Bacon cheeseburger supreme	724	46	57	70

Item	Calories	Total fat (grams)	% total fat	Cholesterol (milli-grams)
JACK IN THE BOX (*cont.*)				
Swiss and bacon burger	643	43	60	99
Ham and Swiss burger	638	39	55	117
Mushroom burger	477	27	51	87
Moby Jack	444	25	51	47
Regular taco	191	11	52	21
Super taco	288	17	53	37
Club pita	284	8	25	43
Chicken supreme	601	36	54	60
Supreme crescent	547	40	66	178
Sausage crescent	584	43	66	187
Pancakes breakfast	626	27	39	85
Scrambled eggs breakfast	719	44	55	260
Breakfast Jack	307	13	38	203
Cooked bacon, 2 slices	70	6	77	10
Chicken strips dinner	689	30	39	100
Shrimp dinner	731	37	48	157
Sirloin steak dinner	699	27	35	75
Cheese nachos	571	35	55	37
Supreme nachos	718	40	50	65
Canadian crescent	472	31	59	226
Pasta seafood salad	394	22	50	48
Taco salad	377	24	57	102
French fries, regular	221	12	49	8
Onion rings	382	23	54	27
Hash-brown potatoes	68	0	0	0
Vanilla shake	320	6	17	25
Strawberry shake	320	7	19	25
Chocolate shake	330	7	19	25
Apple turnover	410	24	53	15

Item	Calories	Total fat (grams)	% total fat	Cholesterol (milli-grams)
KENTUCKY FRIED CHICKEN				
Original recipe				
Wing	181	12	60	67
Side breast	276	17	55	96
Center breast	257	14	49	93
Drumstick	147	9	55	81
Thigh	278	19	62	122
Extra-crispy				
Wing	218	16	66	63
Side breast	354	24	61	66
Center breast	353	21	54	93
Drumstick	173	11	57	65
Thigh	371	26	63	121
Kentucky nuggets, 1	46	3	59	12
Kentucky nugget sauce, 1 oz.				
Barbecue	35	1	26	1
Sweet and sour	58	1	16	1
Honey	49	<1	tr.	1
Mustard	36	1	25	1
Kentucky fries	268	13	44	2
Mashed potatoes w/gravy	62	1	15	1
Mashed potatoes	59	1	15	1
Chicken gravy	59	4	61	2
Buttermilk biscuit	269	14	47	1
Potato salad	141	9	57	11
Baked beans	105	1	9	1
Corn on the cob	176	3	15	1
Cole slaw	103	6	52	4

Item	Calories	Total fat (grams)	% total fat	Cholesterol (milli-grams)
LONG JOHN SILVER'S				
Fish and fries, 3 pieces	853	48	51	106
Fish and fries, 2 pieces	651	36	50	75
Fish and more	978	58	53	88
Fish dinner, 3 pieces	1180	70	53	119
Chicken planks dinner, 3 pieces	885	51	52	25
Chicken planks dinner, 4 pieces	1037	59	51	25
Chicken nuggets dinner, 6 pieces	699	45	58	25
Fish and chicken	935	55	53	56
Seafood platter	976	58	53	95
Clam dinner	955	58	55	27
Batter-fried shrimp dinner	711	45	57	127
Scallop dinner	747	45	54	37
Oyster dinner	789	45	51	55
Kitchen-breaded fish dinner, 3 pieces	940	52	50	101
Kitchen-breaded fish dinner, 2 pieces	818	46	51	76
Fish sandwich platter	835	42	45	75
Seafood salad	426	30	63	113
Ocean chef salad	229	8	31	64
À la carte items				
Batter-fried fish	202	12	53	31
Kitchen-breaded fish	122	6	44	25
Chicken plank	152	8	47	—
Batter-fried shrimp	47	3	57	17
Clam chowder	128	5	35	17
Cole slaw	182	15	74	12

Item	Calories	Total fat (grams)	% total fat	Cholesterol (milli-grams)
LONG JOHN SILVER'S (*cont.*)				
Fries	247	12	44	13
Hush puppies	145	7	43	1
McDONALD'S				
Chicken McNuggets	323	21	59	73
Hamburger	263	11	37	29
Cheeseburger	328	16	44	41
Quarter pounder	427	24	51	81
Quarter pounder w/cheese	525	32	55	107
Big Mac	570	35	55	83
Filet-O-Fish	435	26	54	45
McD.L.T.	680	44	58	101
French fries, regular	220	12	49	9
Biscuit w/sausage, egg	585	40	61	285
Biscuit w/bacon, egg, cheese	483	32	59	263
Sausage McMuffin	427	26	55	59
Sausage McMuffin w/egg	517	33	57	287
Egg McMuffin	340	16	42	259
Hot cakes w/butter, syrup	500	10	18	47
Scrambled eggs	180	13	65	514
Sausage	210	19	81	39
English muffin w/butter	186	15	72	56
Hash brown potatoes	125	7	50	7
Vanilla shake	352	8	20	31
Chocolate shake	383	9	19	30
Strawberry shake	362	9	20	32
Hot fudge sundae	320	9	23	25
Caramel sundae	357	11	28	27

Item	Calories	Total fat (grams)	% total fat	Cholesterol (milligrams)
McDonald's (cont.)				
Apple pie	361	10	25	31
Cherry pie	253	14	49	12
McDonaldland cookies	260	14	48	13
Chocolate chip cookies	308	11	32	10
	342	16	42	18
Wendy's				
Hamburger, multigrain bun	340	7	19	67
Hamburger, white bun	350	18	46	65
Double hamburger, white bun	560	34	55	125
Bacon cheeseburger, white bun	460	28	55	65
Chicken sandwich, multigrain bun	320	10	28	59
Kid's meal hamburger, 2 oz.	220	8	32	20
Chili, 8 oz.	260	8	28	30
French fries, regular	280	14	45	15
Taco salad	390	18	42	40
Frosty dairy dessert	400	14	32	50
Hot stuffed baked potatoes				
Plain	250	2	7	tr.
Sour cream and chives	460	24	47	15
Cheese	590	34	52	22
Chili and cheese	510	20	35	22
Bacon and cheese	570	30	47	22
Broccoli and cheese	500	25	45	22
Ham and cheese omelet	250	17	61	450

Item	Calories	Total fat (grams)	% total fat	Cholesterol (milligrams)
WENDY'S (*cont.*)				
Ham, cheese, mushroom omelet	290	21	65	355
Ham, cheese, onion, and green pepper omelet	280	19	61	525
Mushroom, onion, and green pepper omelet	210	15	64	460
Breakfast sandwich	370	19	46	200
French toast, 2 slices	400	19	43	115
Home fries	360	22	55	20
WHATABURGER				
Whataburger	580	24	37	70
Whataburger, w/cheese	669	33	44	96
Whataburger Jr.	304	14	41	30
Whataburger Jr. w/cheese	351	18	46	42
Justaburger	265	12	41	25
Justaburger w/cheese	312	16	46	37
Whatacatch	475	27	51	34
Whatacatch w/cheese	522	31	53	45
Whataburger double meat	806	41	46	154
Whataburger double meat w/cheese	895	49	49	180
Whatachick'n sandwich	671	32	43	71
French fries, regular	221	12	49	1
French fries, large	332	18	49	1
Onion rings	226	13	52	1
Apple pie	236	12	46	1
Vanilla shake, small	322	9	25	37
Vanilla shake, medium	433	13	27	49

Item	Calories	Total fat (grams)	% total fat	Cholesterol (milli-grams)
WHATABURGER (cont.)				
Vanilla shake, large	647	19	26	74
Vanilla shake, extra large	861	25	26	98
Taquito	310	19	55	223
Taquito w/cheese	357	23	58	235
Egg omelet sandwich	312	15	43	191
Breakfast on a bun	520	34	59	234
Pancakes and sausage, without syrup and butter	407	22	48	77
Pancakes, without syrup and butter	199	3	14	34
Sausage	208	19	82	43
Pecan danish	270	16	53	12
COCA-COLA				
Coca-Cola Classic	144	—	—	—
Coca-Cola	154	—	—	—
Cherry Coke	154	—	—	—
Diet Coke	9	—	—	—
Sprite	142	—	—	—
Mr. Pibb	142	—	—	—
Mello Yello	172	—	—	—
Ramblin' Root Beer	158	—	—	—
Fanta Orange	164	—	—	—
Fanta Grape	168	—	—	—
Fanta Root Beer	158	—	—	—
Fanta Ginger Ale	126	—	—	—
Hi-C Orange	152	—	—	—
Hi-C Lemon	142	—	—	—
Hi-C Punch	154	—	—	—

Item	Calories	Total fat (grams)	% total fat	Cholesterol (milli- grams)
COCA-COLA (*cont.*)				
Hi-C Grape	164	—	—	—
Tab	1	—	—	—
Diet Sprite	3	—	—	—
Minute Maid Orange	160	—	—	—

Sources: Arby's Inc., Atlanta, Georgia; Burger King Corp. Inc.; Church's Fried Chicken, San Antonio, Texas; International Dairy Queen, Inc., Minneapolis, Minnesota; Hardee's Food Systems Inc., Rocky Mount, North Carolina; Jack in the Box Restaurants, Foodmaker, Inc., San Diego, California; Kentucky Fried Chicken Corp., Long John Silvers Inc., Lexington, Kentucky; McDonald's Corp., Oak Brook, Illinois; Wendy's International, Dublin, Ohio; Whataburger Inc., Corpus Christi, Texas; The Coca-Cola Co., Atlanta, Georgia.

Sample Recipes

Fluffy Omelette

4 egg whites
2 egg yolks
1 tablespoon fresh dill, chopped
2 tablespoons skim milk
Salt and pepper to taste
2 teaspoons margarine

Preheat the oven to 400 degrees. In a medium bowl beat the egg whites until stiff, but not dry. In another bowl beat the egg yolks with the milk, salt, pepper, and dill. Fold the beaten egg whites into the yolk mixture. Melt the margarine in a 12-inch skillet with an oven-proof handle. Pour the egg mixture into the skillet and bake in the preheated oven about 12 minutes or until brown and fluffy.

Whole Wheat Blueberry Hotcakes

1 cup whole wheat flour	2 tablespoons brown sugar
1 cup all-purpose flour	1 tablespoon melted margarine
½ teaspoon salt	2 eggs
½ teaspoon baking soda	2¼ cups skim milk
1 tablespoon baking powder	1 cup washed blueberries

Sift the dry ingredients together in a medium mixing bowl. Combine the milk, the melted margarine, and the eggs in another bowl, and mix well. Add the egg mixture to the flour, and stir until smooth. Add the blueberries and mix gently. Spray a nonstick griddle or skillet with cooking spray and place on medium heat. When the griddle is hot, use about ¼ cup of batter for each pancake. Pour the batter onto the heated griddle, and turn when the top of the pancake turns bubbly and the edges become slightly dry.

Breakfast Muesli

3 cups quick-cooking oatmeal	1 teaspoon grated orange rind
2 cups nonfat yogurt	2 grated apples
½ cup slivered almonds	½ cup raisins
1 tablespoon honey	1 cup raspberries

In a medium mixing bowl mix the oats with the nonfat yogurt until moistened. Add the almonds, honey, apples, raisins, and grated orange rind to the yogurt mixture. Allow the oats to soften, about 30 minutes. Just before serving, gently stir in the raspberries.

Cinnamon Pumpkin Waffles

---

1 cup whole wheat flour	½ teaspoon ground nutmeg
2 teaspoons sugar	1½ cups skim milk
½ teaspoon baking soda	2 tablespoons vegetable oil
½ teaspoon baking powder	½ cup canned pumpkin puree
½ tablespoon ground cinnamon	1 egg, separated

Sift dry ingredients together in a medium bowl. Set aside. Combine the milk, pumpkin, oil, and egg yolk in a small bowl, mixing well. Add to the dry mixture gradually, taking care not to overstir. Beat egg white until stiff peaks form, then fold into the pumpkin mixture. Coat a waffle iron with a cooking spray and allow it to preheat. Pour the batter on the heated waffle iron and spread it out to the edge of the iron. Cook until done, 3 to 5 minutes, or until steaming stops. Sprinkle with cinnamon sugar and serve.

Fruity Breakfast Shake

---

2 ripe nectarines, cubed

1 small banana

1 cup nonfat buttermilk

½ cup orange juice

1 tablespoon honey

3 ice cubes, cracked

Combine in a blender all the ingredients except the ice. Blend until smooth. Add the ice and whirl until frothy. Makes two servings.

Whole Wheat Orange Waffles

1 cup whole wheat flour	$\frac{1}{8}$ teaspoon ground cinnamon
$\frac{1}{4}$ cup unprocessed oat bran	1 cup nonfat buttermilk
2 teaspoons baking powder	$\frac{1}{4}$ cup fresh orange juice
$\frac{1}{2}$ teaspoon baking soda	2 tablespoons vegetable oil
$\frac{1}{4}$ teaspoon ground nutmeg	1 egg

Combine the dry ingredients in a medium mixing bowl, stir well, and set aside. Combine buttermilk, orange juice, vegetable oil, and egg in a small mixing bowl, and whisk until well blended. Add to the dry ingredients, stirring until just moistened. Coat a waffle iron with a cooking spray and allow the waffle iron to preheat. Spoon the batter onto the hot waffle iron, spreading the batter to the edges. Bake 3 to 5 minutes or until steaming stops. Repeat with the remaining batter. Serve topped with fresh fruit.

Lunch (or Healthy Brown-Bagging)

Tabbouleh

1 cup bulgur wheat	1 small red onion, diced
2 cups boiling water	1 cup corn, cooked on the cob and then removed from cob
2 ripe tomatoes, diced (reserve the juice)	1 10-oz. can of chick peas, drained and rinsed
1 green bell pepper, diced	Juice of 2 fresh lemons
1 red bell pepper, diced	$\frac{1}{4}$ cup olive oil
1 cup minced fresh parsley	Salt and pepper to taste
$\frac{1}{2}$ cup shredded fresh mint	

Place the bulgur wheat in a medium mixing bowl. Add the boiling water, stir well with fork until wheat is moistened, and let sit for 30 minutes. Place tomatoes and tomato juice, peppers, parsley, mint, red onion, corn, and chick peas in a large serving bowl. Drain the bulgur in a strainer and add to the vegetable mixture. Add the oil and the lemon juice, and toss with a fork. Season with salt and pepper to taste. Cover the bowl with a plastic wrap and refrigerate for an hour or until ready to serve.

Cran-Turkey Sandwich

2 slices whole wheat bread

3 ounces skinless, cooked turkey breast

1 tablespoon whole cranberry sauce

1 ounce Neufchâtel cheese

Mix together the cranberry sauce and the Neufchâtel cheese. Spread the cranberry and cheese mixture on the bread, and add the lettuce and turkey breast. Add an orange for a great brown-bag lunch.

Ziti Salad with Yogurt Dressing

16-ounce package ziti, uncooked

¾ cup nonfat plain yogurt

1 teaspoon curry powder

¼ cup minced fresh parsley

3 tablespoons lemon juice

1 clove garlic, minced

Salt and pepper to taste

1 cucumber, peeled and diced

1 sweet red bell pepper, seeded and chopped

2 medium tomatoes, peeled and chopped

½ cup minced scallions

1 cup frozen corn, thawed

Cook the ziti according to the package directions; drain and set aside. Combine the yogurt, curry powder, parsley, lemon juice, garlic, salt, and pepper in an electric blender and process until smooth. Combine the yogurt sauce and the ziti in a large bowl. Add cucumber, red pepper, tomatoes, scallions, and corn, and toss gently. Cover and chill overnight.

Pita Pocket Salad

1 whole wheat pita bread

½ cup shredded lettuce

½ cup fresh, cleaned spinach

2 slices red onion

4 slices cucumber

2 slices low-fat cheese

½ cup chick peas

2 tomato slices

2 tablespoons low-calorie salad dressing

Split the pita in half, and fill each half with the lettuce, spinach, red onions, cucumbers, cheese, chick peas, and tomato slices. Just before serving, drizzle the salad dressing over the tops of the pockets.

This is a great lunch box sandwich; add the chick peas, tomatoes, and dressing when you sit down to lunch. That way the pita bread won't get soggy.

White Beans and Turkey Chili

2 tablespoon olive oil

2 cloves garlic, minced

½ cup chopped onion

1 teaspoon cumin

1 pound ground lean turkey

1 jalapeño pepper, seeded and chopped (wear rubber gloves)

¼ cup pearl barley

1 10-ounce can chick peas, drained and rinsed

1 10-ounce can cannelli beans, drained and rinsed

6 cups canned low-sodium chicken broth

1 teaspoon dried summer savory

¼ cup minced fresh parsley

Salt

Pepper

2 cups grated low-fat Monterey jack cheese

In a large dutch oven, cook the garlic, onion, and cumin in the olive oil over moderate heat, stirring, until the onions have softened, about 7 minutes. Add the ground turkey, and cook until no longer pink. Add the jalapeño pepper, barley, chick peas, cannelli beans, savory, parsley, and chicken broth. Simmer the mixture, covered, stirring occasionally, for 45 minutes. Season with salt and pepper. Spoon into soup bowls and garnish with the grated cheese.

This chili makes a great take-along lunch, especially during the fall and winter months. Keep it hot in a wide-mouth thermos. Put the grated cheese in a zip-lock sandwich bag and add it to the chili just before you're ready to eat. Some carrot sticks and an apple round out this dish and make it a satisfying, tummy-warming lunch — and one that's high in fiber and low in saturated fats.

Confetti Brown Rice Salad

2 cups cooked brown rice	2 tablespoons fresh lemon juice
½ cup snow peas	1 tablespoon fresh basil, shredded
2 scallions, minced	½ teaspoon dried oregano
½ cup shredded spinach	1 teaspoon Dijon mustard
1 large carrot, diced	1 ripe tomato, cut into wedges
1 tablespoon olive oil	¼ cup minced parsley

In a large salad bowl, combine the brown rice, snow peas, scallions, spinach, and carrot. In a small bowl, whisk together the oil, lemon juice, basil, oregano, and mustard. Toss the dressing with the rice mixture, and garnish the bowl with the tomato wedges and minced parsley.

Finger Lunch

This meal consists of a wide selection of "finger foods," from carrot sticks, raisins, celery sticks, radish roses, and sweet bell pepper strips to cubes of a variety of low-fat cheeses. Dessert could be melon balls, apple wedges, pear pieces, berries, or some homemade quick bread or fruit muffin that travels well. Place each food in its own zip-lock sandwich bag. Add rice cakes or whole wheat crackers to accompany the cheese. This indoor picnic lunch will vary, depending on what you find in your refrigerator and what your child likes the most. Use your imagination to combine a variety of fun foods.

Dinner

Poached Salmon with Zucchini Streamers

4 salmon steaks, about 4 ounces
each

½ cup dry white wine

1 bay leaf

4 peppercorns

1 sprig fresh parsley

1 small onion, sliced

3 medium zucchini

¼ cup shredded fresh basil

Salt and pepper to taste

Vegetable-oil cooking spray

Lemon wedges (optional)

Place the salmon steaks in a large nonreactive skillet, and add the wine, bay leaf, peppercorns, parsley, and onion. Add water to cover and bring to a boil. Reduce the heat and simmer until the salmon flakes easily when tested with a fork, about 8 minutes. Remove from the liquid and set aside. Meanwhile, bring a pot of salted water to a boil. Cut the zucchini into thin, almost transparent strips by using a vegetable peeler. Briefly parboil the zucchini strips in the boiling water until barely tender, 2 to 3 minutes. Drain on a paper towel. Coat a large nonstick skillet with cooking spray, and place over medium-high heat until hot. Add the basil, salt, pepper, and zucchini, and sauté until heated through. Transfer the zucchini strips to a serving plate, and top with the salmon steaks. Garnish with lemon wedges if desired.

A nice side dish for this recipe is steamed carrots with fresh dill. Julienne four large carrots, and steam them in a vegetable steamer until barely tender. In a medium saucepan, melt 2 teaspoons margarine with ¼ cup snipped fresh dill. Add the julienned carrots, toss gently, and serve.

Linguine with Fresh Vegetables

---

8 ounces whole wheat linguine

2 tablespoons olive oil

1 large onion, chopped

3 cloves garlic, minced

1 cup fresh mushrooms, sliced

2 teaspoons dried rosemary

1 tablespoon dried oregano

1 large green bell pepper, seeded and diced

1 large red bell pepper, seeded and diced

1 16-ounce can peeled, whole Italian plum tomatoes

$\frac{1}{4}$ cup chopped cilantro

In a large saucepan, cook the garlic and the onion in the olive oil over medium heat until softened, about 5 minutes. Add the mushrooms, rosemary, oregano, and peppers and cook until softened. Add the tomatoes and simmer, covered, about 30 minutes. While the sauce is simmering, bring a large pot of salted water to a boil. Add the linguine to the water, and bring back to a boil for 5 to 6 minutes or until the linguine is al dente. Drain, place in a large serving bowl, and toss with the sauce. Sprinkle with the chopped cilantro and serve.

Serve this wonderfully filling vegetable linguine with a salad of romaine lettuce, orange segments, and a honey yogurt dressing with poppy seeds as the only accompaniment. Wrap a loaf of a multigrain or whole wheat country bread in foil, and heat it in the oven at 250 degrees for about 15 minutes. For dessert, try apples baked in cider and cinnamon, garnished with vanilla ice milk. Preheat the oven to 350 degrees. Core four baking apples; fill the hollowed core with a mixture of raisins, cinnamon, and chopped walnuts; and sprinkle with some brown sugar. Place in a shallow baking dish and add enough cider to cover the bottom of the dish. Bake, uncovered, 45 minutes to an hour. Serve hot or cold.

Red Snapper in Individual Envelopes

4 6-ounce red snapper fillets
½ pound snow peas, trimmed
2 carrots, julienned
2 scallions, diced

16 fresh mushrooms, whole if small, halved if large
8 lemon slices
Cooking parchment paper or foil

Preheat oven to 400 degrees. Cut the parchment paper into sheets large enough to fold around the fillets. Lay each fillet in the middle of a sheet of parchment paper. Divide the remaining ingredients, and place on the fillets. Close the parchment paper like a package, starting with the top first, closing tightly around the sides, and tucking the ends under. Place the packages on a baking sheet, and bake in the preheated oven for 12 to 15 minutes. Serve in the parchment paper with the brown rice dish that follows.

Brown Rice Apricot Bake

2 teaspoons margarine
1 cup brown rice, uncooked
½ cup chopped onion
¼ cup diced, dried apricots
¼ cup golden raisins

2 cups low-sodium chicken broth
¼ teaspoon curry powder
¼ cup slivered almonds
2 tablespoons chopped parsley
Vegetable-oil cooking spray

Melt the margarine in a large saucepan over medium heat. Add the chopped onion, and cook until tender. Stir in the apricots, raisins, chicken broth, and curry powder. Cover and bring to a boil. Add the rice and remove from the heat. Place the rice mixture in a 1½-quart baking dish coated with cooking spray. Cover, and bake in the oven for 50 minutes, or until the liquid is absorbed. Stir in the slivered almonds and choppd parsley, and garnish with additional parsley sprigs if desired.

Chicken Curry

---

2 stalks celery, chopped
1 medium onion, chopped
1 medium apple, cored and chopped
1 large carrot, chopped
2 cloves garlic, minced
1 teaspoon vegetable-oil cooking spray

1 pound boned chicken breasts, without the skin
1 cup white rice, uncooked
1 tomato, chopped
¼ cup raisins
2 cups low-sodium chicken broth
1 tablespoon curry powder
¼ cup minced fresh parsley

Preheat the oven to 350 degrees. Cook the celery, onion, apple, carrot, and garlic in the oil in a large dutch oven over medium heat until all of the vegetables have softened. Meanwhile, cut the chicken breasts into 1-inch cubes. Add the chicken, rice, tomato, raisins, chicken broth, and curry powder to the dutch oven; bring to a boil; and remove from the heat and cover. Place the covered dutch oven in the preheated oven, and bake 30 minutes, or until the broth is absorbed. Stir in the parsley before serving.

This is a mild curry, best suited to young palates. If your children prefer their food on the spicy side, you can add a touch of red pepper flakes 10 to 15 minutes before the curry is ready.

A nice salad of ripe tomatoes, diced cucumbers, plain yogurt, and fresh dill is very similar to the traditional yogurt side dish that often accompanies all types of curries. Don't forget to pass some mango chutney on the side. For dessert, try a cool, refreshing fruit salad flavored with fragrant fresh mint and honey.

Turkey Loaf

1½ pounds ground turkey

¼ cup minced onion

¾ cup whole wheat bread crumbs

2 egg whites

¼ cup minced celery

1 tablespoon dried savory

2 teaspoons dried marjoram

¼ cup skim milk

1 teaspoon salt

1 teaspoon white pepper

1 clove garlic, minced

¼ cup fresh parsley, chopped

Preheat the oven to 350 degrees. Mix all of the ingredients together well. Form into a loaf, and pack into a lightly oiled 8-by-4-inch bread pan. Bake for about 45 minutes, or until the meat begins to pull away from the sides of pan. Remove from the oven, and let cool for a couple of minutes before cutting.

Ground turkey is a wonderful way to update the old favorite, meatloaf. And unlike regular ground beef and ground pork, ground turkey is very low in fat as well as in cholesterol. Serve this turkey loaf with a refreshing cranberry and orange relish and some boiled red new potatoes and carrots seasoned with fresh dill. Or in keeping with the tradition of meatloaf, serve fresh mashed potatoes spiced up with a mixture of minced garlic, minced parsley, and lemon zest: Cube the potatoes, leaving the skins on, and boil in salted water until done. Mash the potatoes with the minced mixture, and you'll have an old standby with a new flavor twist.

Snacks

Raspberry Banana Flip

1 cup frozen unsweetened raspberries

1 small banana, peeled and cubed

2 cups pineapple juice

$\frac{1}{2}$ cup nonfat yogurt

1 teaspoon honey

3 ice cubes

Sprigs of fresh mint

Blend the raspberries, banana, pineapple juice, yogurt, and honey in a blender until well mixed. Add the ice cubes, and blend until frothy. Garnish with sprigs of fresh mint.

Pumpkin Cranberry Nut Bread

2 cups all-purpose flour

1 cup granulated sugar

1 tablespoon pumpkin pie spice

1 teaspoon baking soda

$\frac{1}{2}$ teaspoon salt

2 eggs, lightly beaten

1 tablespoon grated orange rind

1 16-ounce can solid-pack pumpkin

$\frac{1}{2}$ cup vegetable oil

1 cup cranberries, coarsely chopped

$\frac{1}{2}$ cup walnuts, coarsely chopped

Preheat the oven to 350 degrees. In a large mixing bowl, combine the flour, sugar, pumpkin pie spice, baking soda, and salt, and set aside. In a medium bowl, combine the eggs, grated orange rind, pumpkin, and oil. Add the liquid ingredients to the dry ingredients, and stir until just moistened. Fold in the cranberries and the walnuts. Spoon the batter into an oiled and floured 9-by-5-inch loaf pan. Bake in the preheated oven for 45 to 50 minutes, or until a toothpick comes out clean. (This bread is also great in the mornings toasted.)

Fruit Kabobs

Fresh strawberries, washed and hulled

Melon balls, any variety

Fresh kiwis, peeled and cubed

Fresh pineapple, cubed

Fresh apricots, halved

Red flame grapes, washed

Juice of one lemon

1 tablespoon honey

Mix the lemon juice and honey in a small bowl, and set aside. Thread the fruit alternately on 6-inch wooden skewers. Place the kabobs on a platter, and drizzle the lemon and honey over them. Chill covered until ready to eat.

This is a great snack that kids can put together themselves once the ingredients are arranged.

Winter Fruit Compote

8 ounces dried apricots

4 ounces dried peaches

4 ounces dried nectarines

1 orange, sliced

3 slices fresh lemon

2 whole cloves

Place the dried fruit, lemon and orange slices, and cloves in a large saucepan. Cover the fruit mixture with cold water, place a lid on the pan, and simmer 40 to 45 minutes, or until tender. The fruit compote may be sweetened with a little brown sugar if desired. Serve warm or cold. It's delicious with some plain, nonfat yogurt spooned over the top.

In place of the lemon and orange, you can flavor the compote with preserved or candied ginger or half a vanilla bean. This dried compote is also wonderful without any flavoring other than the fruit itself.

Lemon Drop Cookies

2 cups all-purpose flour

1 tablespoon plus 1 teaspoon baking powder

$\frac{1}{4}$ teaspoon salt

$\frac{1}{4}$ cup of margarine, softened

1 cup sugar

2 tablespoons poppy seeds

2 eggs

2 tablespoons grated lemon rind

$\frac{1}{4}$ cup fresh lemon juice

Cooking spray

Preheat the oven to 350 degrees. Combine the flour, baking powder, and salt in a small mixing bowl, and set aside. Cream the margarine in a medium bowl until light and fluffy. Little by little, add the sugar, beating well after each addition. Add the poppy seeds, eggs, lemon rind, and lemon juice, and beat well. Add the flour mixture, and stir until blended, but do not overmix. Drop the dough by heaping teaspoonfuls onto cookie sheets that have been lightly dusted with the cooking spray. Bake for 10 minutes in the preheated oven, or until the edges of the cookies just begin to brown. Cool slightly on the cookie sheets, and then place on a wire rack to complete the cooling.

Fruits and vegetables are among the best snacks for your child. "Snack food" such as potato chips tends to be high in fats and sodium. Some of the better choices among snack foods are salt-free Dutch-style hard pretzels and air-popped popcorn. Having a ready supply of fresh or dried fruits on hand, as well as carrot and celery sticks crisping in water in the refrigerator, makes munching a healthy proposition.

Heart Glossary Terms

Adipose: Fat, or fatty in nature.

Aerobic exercise: Repetitive, rhythmic exercise that requires oxygen from the air for the muscles to continue to work and requires heart and breathing (cardiorespiratory) effort. Examples are running, swimming, cycling, and jumping rope.

Amino acids: Simple organic compounds that are the building blocks of proteins. Examples include leucine and tryptophan.

Angina pectoris: Literally, "chest pain." It is a feeling of pressing or "tight" pain in the middle of the chest, sometimes traveling into the left arm. It is caused by lack of enough oxygen to the heart muscle, brought on by exertion and relieved by rest or nitroglycerin placed under the tongue.

Angiography: An X ray procedure that gives a detailed picture of the arteries, such as the coronary arteries of the heart. A dye is injected into the artery through a flexible tube (a catheter), and the dye shows up on the X ray. In coronary angiography, the catheter is inserted into the femoral artery in the groin and is threaded up through the left ventricle of the heart into the beginning of the aorta, and into the openings of the coronary arteries. The purpose is to detect significant blockage.

Angioplasty (coronary-artery balloon angioplasty): A procedure, not requiring open-heart surgery, used to unblock coronary arteries. A thin and flexible tube that holds an uninflated balloon is inserted into the blocked artery. The balloon is then inflated, and the blockage is crushed down.

Aorta: The main artery of the body, which arises from the left ventricle of the heart and carries oxygen and nutrients throughout the entire system except to the lungs (which are fed by the pulmonary arteries).

Apolipoprotein A1 (ApoA1): The major apolipoprotein of HDL, which facilitates the removal of cholesterol from the surface of cells, or the linings of arteries, for transport back to the liver. Having too little ApoA1 increases the risk of coronary heart disease and may explain the occurrence of early coronary heart disease in the presence of normal blood cholesterol levels.

Apolipoprotein B (ApoB): The major protein of LDL, which is picked up by LDL receptors present on liver and nonliver cells. These receptors admit LDL into the liver cells (lowering its level in the blood), where it is broken down into cholesterol and amino acids, which are then used by the cells. In familial hyperlipidemia (FH), or as a result of excessive saturated fat or cholesterol in the diet, these receptors will be fewer or the less active. As a result, less LDL leaves the blood to enter the cells, and the LDL level rises in the blood. Having too much ApoB (hyperapo-B-lipoproteinemia) may explain early coronary heart disease in the presence of normal cholesterol levels.

Apolipoproteins: Special proteins in the blood that combine with lipids, such as cholesterol or triglyceride to form lipoproteins.

Arteriosclerosis: Literally, "hardening of the arteries." This is a broad term, including atherosclerosis.

Atherosclerosis: A form of arteriosclerosis in which a gradual and progressive narrowing of the arteries by plaque interferes with the blood's delivery of oxygen and other nutrients. In the arteries of the heart or the coronary arteries, atherosclerosis may lead to angina pectoris or a heart attack.

Bile acid-binding agents (see *cholestyramine* and *colestipol*): Drugs used to lower blood LDL levels. They are not absorbed into the blood but bind bile acids in the intestine to eliminate them in the stool. To make up for the loss of bile acids, the liver is forced to use up its own cholesterol and to pull LDL out of the blood to replace the used-up cholesterol.

Blood cholesterol: All the cholesterol in the blood is in the form of lipoproteins. Some are manufactured in the liver, and some come from the diet. Cholesterol is carried throughout the body for normal function. Excess levels lead to the development of atherosclerosis and, in the heart, to coronary heart disease.

Blood pressure: The force of the blood against the walls of the arteries, created by the pumping action of the heart as it propels blood throughout the body. *Systolic blood pressure* is the first or higher number in a blood pressure reading. It is the pressure present at the end of the heart's contracting. *Diastolic blood pressure* is the second or lower number in a blood pressure reading. It is the pressure when the heart relaxes between contractions.

Bogalusa Heart Study: A large and valuable ongoing study of many children in Louisiana, begun in the 1970s to clarify the beginnings and development of atherosclerosis. Special emphasis has been placed on the role of diet and blood cholesterol levels. We would like to regard these studies as applying the contributions of the Framingham Heart Study on adults to the entire concept of bringing prevention to all of our children.

Bran: A type of fiber, which is the skin or husk of various grains, such as oat, barley, rye, and wheat.

Calorie: A unit of heat (energy) that is required to raise the temperature of 1 gram of water by 1 degree centigrade. Calories are supplied by carbohydrates (4 calories per gram), by proteins (also 4 calories per gram), and by fat (9 calories per gram).

Carbohydrates: One of the three basic nutrients (the others are protein and fat) that supply energy (calories) to the body. Each gram of carbohydrate provides 4 calories. There are two basic kinds of carbohydrate: simple carbohydrate (sugars) and complex carbohydrate (starches and fiber).

Cardiovascular disease: An ailment of the heart and/or the blood vessels, often caused by atherosclerosis.

Cerebral: Pertaining to the brain.

Cholesterol: A soft wax found only in animal cells. It is not a fat. In order to be soluble in blood, it needs to combine with protein to become a lipoprotein. The body is capable of making all the cholesterol it needs for normal body functions, which includes making cell membranes, hormones, bile acid, and vitamin D.

Cholestyramine: A bile acid-binding drug used to lower LDL. Normally, about 70 percent of the LDL removed from the blood is removed by the liver via its LDL receptors. This drug interferes with (binds) the return of bile acids from the intestine to the liver, so that the liver must use up much more of its own cholesterol for the manufacture of more bile acids. Depleted of its own cholesterol and needing more, the liver has to pull more LDL out of the blood to make these bile acids. The net result is a lowering of blood total and LDL cholesterol.

Chylomicron: A lipoprotein that transports dietary triglyceride and cholesterol from the intestine into the bloodstream.

Colestipol: A bile acid-binding drug, similar to cholestyramine in its action and used to lower LDL. It has less bulk than cholestyramine but does not have as good a taste, texture, or smell.

Complex carbohydrate: Starch and fiber that come from plants. When substituted for saturated fat in the diet, they help to lower blood cholesterol. Starch is found in cereals, breads, pasta, rice, lima beans, corn, and dried beans and peas.

Coronary angiography: See *angiography*.

Coronary arteries: The blood vessels (three major ones) that carry oxygen and nutrients to the heart muscle. Their narrowing by atherosclerosis is called *coronary artery disease*, which may damage the heart muscle and lead to pain (angina pectoris) or a heart attack.

Coronary artery bypass: An open-heart operation in which a portion of a leg vein (the saphenous vein) is used to connect the aorta with a coronary artery beyond the area where it has been blocked by atherosclerosis, in essence "bypassing" the obstructed portion of artery. A "triple bypass" uses grafts to bypass three blocked arteries.

Dietary cholesterol: In the foods you eat, and only those of animal origin, dietary cholesterol, along with saturated fat, tends to raise blood cholesterol levels. Excess dietary cholesterol increases the risk of heart disease.

Epidemiology: The study of a disease as it affects different populations, and the factors that enter into the differences.

Familial: Hereditary or genetic; affecting the individual members of a family.

Familial hypercholesterolemia (FH): An uncommon form of high cholesterol levels that is genetic. The most common form, occurring in about 1 in 500 children, is heterozygous, the result of a single dominant gene passed down from one parent. Cholesterol levels are usually over 250, and LDL levels are proportionately high. If the gene is passed down from both parents, it is call *homozygous*. This is a rare condition, occurring in only about 1 in 1 million. These children have sky-high total cholesterol levels, often over 1,000, and a similarly high LDL level. These children often have fatty deposits apparent on the skin and around their corneas. They are at high risk for early heart attack or stroke. They are usually resistant to dietary management alone, requiring drug or even more aggressive therapy.

Fat: One of the three basic nutrients (the others are protein and carbohydrate) that supply energy (calories) to the body. There are three types of fats: saturated, monounsaturated, and polyunsaturated. A gram of every kind of fat provides 9 calories. Besides providing energy, fat is required for normal body function, such as the absorption of some vitamins.

Fatty acids: The basic chemical building blocks of fats, which may be saturated, monounsaturated, or polyunsaturated. All dietary fats are a mixture of the three types of fatty acids in varying amounts.

Fatty streak: The earliest form of atherosclerosis, when cholesterol and fatty materials are deposited within the walls of the arteries. At this stage, the deposits are flat, so they do not yet block the flow of blood through the arteries.

Fiber: An indigestible vegetable material, usually low in calories. There are two kinds: water-soluble fiber (found in oat bran, apples, oranges, and dried beans), which helps lower blood cholesterol levels, and water-insoluble fiber (such as in wheat bran), which has no effect on cholesterol levels.

Fibrous plaque: An intermediate form of atherosclerosis in which collections of materials (cholesterol, fibrous tissue, clotted blood, and calcium) accumulate on the lining walls of the arteries and begin to narrow the arterial openings.

Framingham Heart Study: An epidemiological research project on heart disease carried out in Massachusetts since 1948, providing hundreds of valuable, carefully controlled studies of risk factors and prevention factors, such as control of hypertension and cholesterol, which have been widely followed.

Gram (g): A metric unit of weight in which dietary fat, carbohydrate, and protein are usually shown on food labels. One gram of protein and carbohydrate each provides 4 calories of energy. One gram of fat provides 9 calories. There are just over 28 grams in 1 ounce by weight.

Heart attack: A term that generally refers to the death of a part of the heart muscle (myocardial infarction), usually caused by the closing off of a coronary artery branch as the result of progressive coronary-artery atherosclerosis. It is usually accompanied by chest pain, but at times it may occur without pain (a silent heart attack).

Heart valves: Flexible structures that permit the flow of blood in only one direction. If the opening is too small, the condition is called *stenosis*, as in *mitral stenosis*. If the opening is too large, the condition is called *insufficiency*, as in *tricuspid insufficiency*. The heart has four valves: the mitral valve, for the passage of blood from the left atrium to the left ventricle; the tricuspid valve, for the passage of blood from the right atrium to the right ventricle; the aortic valve, for passage of blood from the left ventricle into the aorta; and the pulmonary valve, for passage of blood from the right ventricle into the pulmonary artery.

Heterozygous: In a hereditary disease, a person who carries one normal gene and one abnormal gene is heterozygous for that disease. A person with one faulty gene (for LDL receptors) is called an *FH* (familial hypercholesterolemia) *heterozygote*. This condition exists in about 1 in 500 children, and this child will have a cholesterol level of about 300. Half of such children, if untreated, develop coronary heart disease by age forty in males and by age fifty in females.

High-density lipoprotein (HDL): HDLs carry a small amount of cholesterol and carry cholesterol away from the cells and tissues (such as artery walls) and back to the liver for excretion from the body. Therefore, the higher the HDL level, the better. Low levels increase the risk of coronary heart disease. HDLs are referred to as *good cholesterol*.

Homozygous: In a hereditary disease, a person who carries both genes for the disease is homozygous for that disease. In familial hypercholesterolemia (FH), the person is called an *FH homozygote*. This condition occurs in only about 1 in 1 million children, and this child will have a cholesterol level of about 1,000. Untreated, such children often develop coronary heart disease before the age of twenty, and many die before that age.

Hydrogenation: A chemical process that changes liquid vegetable oils that are unsaturated into more saturated solid fat. This process is used to increase the shelf life of a product, even though the saturated fat is less healthy. Many commercial products contain hydrogenated vegetable oil, so you need to read the labels.

Hypercholesterolemia: A high level of total cholesterol in the blood.

Hyperlipidemia: A high level of both total cholesterol and triglyceride in the blood.

Hypertension: High blood pressure; excessive pressure of the blood within the arteries.

Intima: The innermost layer, or lining, of an artery. It is here that deposits of atherosclerotic plaque begin to block the opening of the artery, interfering with the free passage of blood.

LDL receptors: Proteins on the surface of cells that allow LDL to be taken into the cells for use. The fewer the receptors or the less they do their job, the more the LDL accumulates in the blood, thereby raising blood cholesterol levels. This condition occurs with too much dietary saturated fat and cholesterol, and in hereditary conditions.

Lesion: An abnormal defect or loss of function in a body part. A focal lesion is one with definite limits within a small area.

Lipid: A fat or fatlike substance, insoluble in water, such as cholesterol or triglyceride. Lipids are present in the blood and in other body tissues.

Lipid profile: A blood test that breaks down total cholesterol into its component parts: LDL cholesterol, HDL cholesterol, and triglyceride or VLDL cholesterol. The test requires blood from a vein after a 12-hour fast. Total cholesterol = LDL + HDL + VLDL (or triglyceride ÷ 5).

Lipoproteins: A combination of proteins (called *apolipoproteins*) with lipids (such as cholesterol or triglyceride) that makes a soluble package that can be transported through the blood for use throughout the body. These packages are classified according to their density.

Low-density lipoprotein (LDL): LDL is 50 percent cholesterol and is responsible for depositing cholesterol inside the artery walls. Therefore, the lower the LDL level, the better. High levels increase the risk of coronary heart disease. LDL is referred to as *bad cholesterol*.

Milligram (mg): A metric unit of weight equal to .001 gram (1,000 mg equal 1 gram). Cholesterol amounts in foods and levels in the blood are expressed in milligrams.

Monounsaturated fat: A type of fat, liquid at room temperature, that has little effect on raising or lowering blood cholesterol, except by replacing saturated fat in the diet. It is found in olive oil, peanut oil, and canola (rapeseed) soil.

Myocardial infarction: An area of death in the heart muscle due to the loss of circulation through a branch of the coronary artery. This is the end result of a progressive closure of the artery by the process of atherosclerosis.

Necrosis: Death of a circumscribed portion of tissue. It occurs in a part of the brain in a stroke or in a portion of heart muscle in a myocardial infarction.

Niacin (nicotinic acid): A B vitamin that, when used in high doses, is a cholesterol-reducing drug. It acts by reducing the liver's production of VLDL. Because it often has side effects when used in therapeutic doses, it should be used only in selected cases and under the guidance of a physician.

Olestra: A fat replacer, introduced in 1990 by Procter & Gamble. Made from triglyceride, it reduces calories across the board and does not affect taste or texture. It is not hydrolyzed or absorbed by the body. Blended with vegetable oils, it can be cooked or baked to produce snack foods, such as potato or corn chips.

Omega-3 fatty acid (fish oil): A type of polyunsaturated fat found in fish in varying amounts, especially in fatty fish, that helps to lower blood cholesterol levels.

Open-heart surgery: An operation performed on a heart while the patient's blood is diverted through a heart–lung machine. The surgery may be performed on the heart walls, on the valves, or on the coronary arteries.

Peripheral vascular disease: A progressive disease process in which the leg arteries are narrowed by atherosclerosis, impairing their circulation of blood to the limbs below the areas of blockage.

Polyunsaturated fat: A type of fat, liquid at room temperature, that does help lower blood cholesterol. It is found mostly in plant foods, including safflower, sunflower, corn, and soybean oils.

Protein: One of the three basic nutrients (the others are carbohydrate and fat) that supply energy (calories) to the body. Each gram of protein provides 4 calories. Protein is an essential nutrient, becoming a part of all tissues of the body, including muscle, bone, skin, and blood.

Saturated fat: A fat found in food mainly of animal origin, but also in products made from palm and coconut oil. It raises blood cholesterol more than anything else in the diet. It is found in the marbling and on the edges of meat, in whole milk and whole-milk products, and in the skin of poultry. It is a white, oily substance that is solid at room temperature.

Simplesse: A fat replacer made from egg whites and milk protein and introduced in 1990 by the Nutrasweet Division of Monsanto. Because it cannot be used in cooking, it is found in frozen desserts, such as Simple Pleasures. Introduced with enthusiasm by its originator, it has not met with universal acclaim as a taste sensation. Improved modifications of the original formula can be expected in the future.

Step One Diet: Diet recommended by the American Heart Association, which recommends this distribution of the calories in the diet:

Total fat	30%
Saturated fat	10%
Polyunsaturated fat	10%
Monounsaturated fat	10–5%
Cholesterol	300 mg per day
Carbohydrate	50%–60%
Protein	10–20%

Step Two Diet: A stricter diet for lowering total cholesterol and LDL cholesterol levels. The total fat, carbohydrate, and protein levels are the same as in the Step One diet. The different recommendations are:

| Saturated fat | Less than 7% |
| Cholesterol | Less than 200 mg per day |

Stroke: Also referred to as a *cerebrovascular accident*; the sudden loss of blood circulation to a circumscribed part of the brain, resulting from a clot forming in a cerebral artery branch (a cerebral thrombosis), from a clot arriving in a cerebral artery from elsewhere (a cerebral embolism), or from the rupture of a cerebral artery (a cerebral hemorrhage). A stroke is often the result of cerebral atherosclerosis or hypertension.

Thrombosis: The formation of a blood clot that partially or completely blocks a blood vessel, such as coronary or cerebral thrombosis.

Total fat: The sum of the saturated, monounsaturated, and polyunsaturated fat present in food.

Tracking: The observed phenomenon that if the blood cholesterol level is found to be elevated in early childhood, there is a tendency for it to remain high as the child grows older. Its importance lies in its predictability, which provides us with the opportunity to identify children at possible risk and to take measures to reduce this risk.

Transmonounsaturated fatty acids: Products of the hydrogenation of margarines (in order to make them firmer) that act like saturated fat to raise blood cholesterol levels. The harder the margarine, the more transmonounsaturated fatty acids it contains.

Triglyceride: A type of lipid found in the blood and tissues of the body. It is made in the liver and is also found in the diet. Most of the body's fat stores are triglycerides, but too much triglyceride in the blood increases the risk of heart disease.

Unsaturated fat: A clear, oily substance, usually liquid at room temperature. The two main types are monounsaturated and polyunsaturated.

Vascular: Pertaining to the blood vessels.

Very-low-density lipoprotein (VLDL): A lipoprotein made in the liver that is the main carrier of triglyceride, as well as of some cholesterol. Some of the broken-down remnants of VLDL are converted into the cholesterol-rich LDL.

Recommended Readings

Do you want to read more? I can recommend the following books to you:

CHAPTER 1

Peter Kwiterovich, *Beyond Cholesterol*. Baltimore: Johns Hopkins University Press, 1989.

Robert Kowalski, *Cholesterol and Children*. New York: Harper & Row, 1988.

"Hyperlipidemia in Childhood and the Development of Atherosclerosis," *Annals of the New York Academy of Sciences*, 1991.

CHAPTER 4

Dr. Dean Ornish's Program for Reversing Heart Disease. New York: Random House, 1991.

Judith Pacht, *Lean or Lavish*. New York: Warner Books, 1991.

CHAPTER 8

Kenneth Cooper, *Controlling Cholesterol*. New York: Bantam Books, 1988.

American Heart Association, *Low-Fat, Low-Cholesterol Cookbook*. New York: Times Books, 1989.

The Reader's Digest Guide to Family Fitness. Write to Reprint Editor, *Reader's Digest*, Pleasantville, NY 10570.

Know Your Body. Write to the American Health Foundation, 320 East 43rd Street, New York, NY 10017.

Index

Cake *(cont.)*
  oat-bran, 164
  saturated fat content, 232–233,
    235–236, 237, 239
Calcium
  dietary sources, 44–45, 89
  recommended daily allowance, 45
Calories
  average daily expenditure, 71–73
  average daily requirements, 71–
    72
  carbohydrate-based, 40, 74, 79
  definition, 287
  fat-based, 40, 73, 74
  calculation of, 106–107, 181
  protein-based, 40, 74
Camp food, 135, 137–138
Camps, weight-loss, 173
Candy
  calorie content, 229–232
  cholesterol content, 229–232
  fat content, 229–232
  no-fat, 100
  saturated fat content, 229–232
Canned foods
  fish and shellfish, 111, 114, 211–
    212, 213, 214, 215
  fruits, 114, 182, 183, 184, 185
  shopping for, 114–115
  vegetables, 114, 187, 188, 189,
    191, 192
Canola oil, 49, 65, 99, 108, 115,
  226
Carbohydrates
  as calorie source, 47
  complex, 48, 288
  definition, 287
  as percentage of total diet, 40,
    74, 79

Cardiovascular disease. *See also*
  Heart disease
  definition, 287
Casseroles. *See* Combination dishes
Castelli, William T., v–vii
Centers for Disease Control, 178
Cereals
  bran, 61–62, 98, 195
  calorie content, 195–198
  cholesterol content, 195–198
  fat content, 113–114, 195–198
  fiber content, 63, 113
  in low-fat diet, 61–62, 63
  with nuts, 98
  oat-bran, 98, 196, 197
  saturated fat content, 195–198
  shopping for, 113–114
  sugar content, 97, 113–114
  whole-grain, 124
Cheese
  American, 89, 221
  as calcium source, 89
  calorie content, 221–223
  cholesterol content, 58, 221–223
  fat content, 221–223
  low-fat, 58–59, 83, 90, 112
  Mozzarella, 59, 89, 221, 223
  nonfat, 90
  as protein source, 89
  recommended weekly servings, 89
  saturated fat content, 221–223
Chicken
  calorie content, 216–217
  cholesterol content, 216–217
  fast-food, 125, 126
    Burger King, 127
    Hardee's, 130–131
    Kentucky Fried Chicken, 129,
      261